MOTHERS AND ILLICIT DRUGS:
TRANSCENDING THE MYTHS

During the past decade, media and medical forces have combined to create an alarming view of pregnant mothers who use illicit drugs. The result has been increased state control of these women and their infants. This in-depth study is the first in Canada to look at how mothers who use illicit drugs regard the laws, medical practices, and social services that intervene in their lives.

Focusing on practices in western Canada, Susan C. Boyd argues that licit and illicit drug categories are artificial and dangerous and that the evidence for neonatal syndrome (NAS) is suspect and ideologically driven. She shows that women of colour and poor women are treated much more harshly by authorities, that current regulations erode women's civil liberties, and that social control is the aim of drug policy and law. The study highlights mothers' views of the NAS program at Sunny Hill Hospital for Children in Vancouver.

Writing from a critical feminist perspective, Boyd exposes some surprising social fictions – those that separate 'good' and 'bad' drugs, as they do 'good' and 'bad' mothers.

SUSAN C. BOYD is Assistant Professor, School of Criminology, Simon Fraser University.

SUSAN C. BOYD

Mothers and Illicit Drugs: Transcending the Myths

UNIVERSITY OF TORONTO PRESS
Toronto Buffalo London

© University of Toronto Press Incorporated 1999
Toronto Buffalo London
Printed in Canada

ISBN 0-8020-4331-3 (cloth)
ISBN 0-8020-8151-7 (paper)

Canadian Cataloguing in Publication Data

Boyd, Susan C., 1953–
    Mothers and illicit drugs : transcending the myths

    Includes bibliographic references and index
    ISBN 0-8020-4331-3 (bound)   ISBN 0-8020-8151-7 (pbk.)

    1. Mothers – Drug use – Canada.   2. Mothers – Drug use –
    United States.   I. Title.

    HV5824.W6B69 1999   362.29′085′2   C98-931829-X

University of Toronto Press acknowledges the financial assistance to its publishing program of the Canada Council for the Arts and the Ontario Arts Council.

This book has been published with the help of a grant from the Humanities and Social Sciences Federation of Canada, using funds provided by the Social Sciences and Humanities Research Council of Canada.

This book is dedicated to my children, Jade and Iain Boyd.

Contents

Acknowledgments

Without the participation of all the women interviewed for this book, it would have been impossible to write. Their contribution was invaluable. I am also grateful to my supervisory committee – Bruce Alexander, Neil Boyd, Dorothy Chunn, and Karlene Faith – at Simon Fraser University, whose comments, direction, and support contributed to this work.

I would also like to thank Ann Brainer for her patience and computer expertise in formatting this book; and Cheryl Anderson, Starla Anderson, Penny Mumm, and Theresa MacDonald for their proof-reading and unfailing encouragement. I would also like to thank Irit Shimrat and Beverley Beetham Endersby for their excellent copy-editing skills.

I am indebted to the Social Sciences and Humanities Research Council of Canada, Canadian Soroptomist, and Simon Fraser University; without their assistance this project might not have been completed. As well, I am grateful to the Humanities and Social Sciences Federation of Canada, who provided funding through the Social Sciences and Humanities Research Council of Canada. I would also like to thank Virgil Duff of University of Toronto Press for his interest and support in the publication of this book.

Finally, I wish to thank my many friends and family members for their support all these years, and for providing me with the spirit to keep going. I am especially grateful to Gloria Watkins, Carolyn Crichton, and Otis LeBlond, whose loving friendship and support have sustained me. I wish to acknowledge my mother, Catherine Boyd, and all of my brothers and sisters, Diana, Jean, Robert, Tommy, Eddie, Howard, and my sister-in-law Suzanne, who have encouraged me. A special thanks to my two children, Jade Boyd and Iain Boyd, who continue to inspire me.

MOTHERS AND ILLICIT DRUGS:
TRANSCENDING THE MYTHS

1

A Gender Analysis

Since the mid-1980s the mass media and many members of the medical profession have demonized expectant mothers who use illicit drugs, viewing them as unfit parents who damage their unborn children through their continued drug use. The image created to convey this message is a familiar one: We see a white male doctor holding a premature infant – a separate entity from the mother – and often we are informed that the child is suffering from withdrawal symptoms which may include tremors, a high-pitched cry, and arching of the back, and that such infants are severely damaged, creating a new underclass of children who will be a drain on social services, the medical community, and even the criminal justice system.

Since the 1980s, social science research in the area of illicit drug use has undergone a shift in focus – from female illicit drug users to the developing foetuses of women who use illicit drugs. Maternal drug use; assessment of risk; and the identification, regulation, treatments, and control of wayward mothers and their infants have become central concerns in conservative and liberal research on illicit drug use. However, neither conservative nor liberal paradigms offer solutions for underlying problems associated with class, gender, and race. In addition, the negative impact of the medical and social service professions, and of drug legislation, on women who use illicit drugs and on their infants is ignored.

This book provides a view of women who use illicit narcotics in Canada, focusing on their opinions regarding the law, medical and social service policy, and regulations that affect their lives, against the background of the social control of women in Western society. Specifically, it brings forward the opinions of mothers who use illicit drugs concerning the medical treatment of adult women and their newborn infants, the cultural construction of neonatal abstinence syndrome (NAS), Canadian narcotics laws, and the effects of drug treatments, in addition to providing data on the role of social services in relation to intervention and to the apprehension of children.

This book also undertakes a feminist analysis of the literature on and explores society's attitudes towards mothers and illicit drug use. It is based on a study which included open-ended interviews with mothers in Western Canada in 1993–4. Aside from having in common their status as mothers and their use of illicit drugs, the women interviewed did not form a homogeneous group, but were diverse in race, class, and age. This was the first in-depth study in Canada focusing on how mothers who use illicit drugs view the agencies of law, social services, and the medical profession. Rather than focus on victimization and the risks and harms associated with individual drug use, this work examines women's agency and legal and socio-economic factors that shape drug use.

This book is informed by the work of early critical researchers who literally transformed the study of illicit drug use in the 1960s (Becker, 1963; Gusfield, 1963; Lindesmith, 1965; Schur, 1962; Winick, 1962). The movement away from perceiving the 'addict' as a criminal and towards an examination of how legal and social conventions define the illicit drug user, both symbolically and directly, stems from their research. Later research, both Canadian and U.S. (Alexander & Hadaway, 1981; Blackwell, 1983; Boyd, 1983, 1984; Brecher & The Editors of *Consumer Reports*, 1972; Judson, 1973; Morgan, 1978, 1983; Preble & Casey, 1969; Reinarman, 1979; Small, 1978; Szasz, 1974; Trebach, 1982; Waldorf, 1973; Waldorf & Biernacki, 1979; Weil, 1972; Zinberg, Harding, & Apsler, 1978), continued to examine the social construction of the line dividing licit and illicit drugs and the impact of morality, law, race, and class in defining illicit drug use in North America.

Critical researchers acknowledge that 'crime' is a political construct, where the state can choose to act, or fail to act, and where selective criminalization takes place (Tunnell, 1993). In North America the most dangerous drugs are legal. Tobacco and alcohol are more lethal than the more benign illicit drugs, such as marijuana, and both heroin and cocaine (Alexander, 1990; Boyd, 1991; Trebach, 1987; Weil & Rosen, 1993). The so-called dangers of illicit drugs are widely depicted by both government and the media. But the real dangers of legal drugs, including alcohol, tobacco, and pharmaceuticals, are viewed differently.

Currently, illicit drug use is perceived as deviant behaviour, and the selective criminalization of women who use illicit drugs in North America is obscured by the use of labels such as 'addict' and 'drug baby.' The word 'addict' has only recently developed as a negative label reserved for illicit drug users (Alexander, 1990). Imprecise definitions and language have led to misleading information about infants exposed to maternal drug use and people who use both legal and illegal drugs. This book attempts to demystify the labels applied to women who use illicit drugs, and their infants, for, as Faith states,

> when we recognize the contextual bases of illegal actions and the discriminatory nature of criminalization processes as applied to either men or women, and when we demystify labelled women by showing their diversities as well as the commonalities they share as women in a gendered power structure, we lose the need for labels, or for gendered stereotypes. (1993, p. 59)

This book examines the fallacy of the 'threat of drugs,' and proposes that 'social control' has been, and continues to be, a central concept of analysis adopted by researchers examining the criminalization of specific drugs in North America and, more recently, when examining maternal drug use.

The term 'social control' is appealing because it can be utilized as a conceptual tool when analysing relations between the powerful and powerless (Edwards, 1988). In addition, the term gives a theoretical unity to a wide range of social institutions and practices (Edwards, 1988). All social measures which manage, contain, punish, repress, direct, or redirect individuals or groups are forms of social control (Edwards, 1988). Cohen refers to social control as 'the organized ways in which society responds to behaviour and people it regards as deviant, problematic, worrying, threatening, troublesome or undesirable in some way or another' (1985, p. 1). Social control can be direct and explicit or indirect and implicit.

Women and Social Control

Feminists have noted and challenged specific sites of regulation and social control that are ignored by both critical and non-critical researchers. These sites are gender-specific, centring on familial ideology[1] and biological reproduction as the loci of social regulation. Smart and Smart note that women experience social control in relation to their reproductive cycles, double standards of morality, social and legal subordination, the separation of the public and private spheres – an ideology that relegates a woman's place to the private sphere (1978, p. 3). However, the public/ private divide is ideological and 'indeterminate and shifting' (Boyd, 1997,

p. 4). This book links the research on reproductive autonomy and familial ideology with critical analysis of drug use in Western society.

Women are regulated outside of the criminal justice system through medical (Clarke, 1996) and social service policy (Maher, 1992). Both professions have incorporated assumptions about women's role in society. Women who do not conform to familial ideology are regulated and punished. The law also becomes an integral part of the regulation of women in the areas of medicine and social services by appropriating their categorizations and practices into its domain (Smart, 1989, p. 96).

Women and Illicit Drug Use

Although women who use illicit drugs are subject to social control and arrest for drug-related offences (the possession of narcotics is a criminal offence in Canada and many other Western nations), little research had been done about women who used illicit drugs. The majority of studies (except for Blackwell, 1983; Erickson, Adlaf, Murray, & Smart, 1987; Waldorf, Reinarman, & Murphy, 1991) focused on men's perceptions of illicit drug use (Addiction Research Foundation, 1994; Reed, 1987).

Until recently, there was little feminist response to critical research on illicit drug use. Early literature on female drug users centred on the legal use of medically prescribed drugs and on multinational pharmaceutical companies (Cooperstock & Hill, 1982; Lexchin, 1984; McDonnell, 1986; Penfold & Walker, 1983). Women are prescribed more pharmaceutical drugs than are men (Ettorre, 1992; Lexchin, 1984; McDonnell, 1986; Penfold & Walker, 1983), and most of these drugs are related to their reproductive capacity (McDonnell, 1986, p. 4). Women also consume more legal psychoactive drugs than do men (Addiction Research Foundation, 1994). Like Cooperstock and Hill (1982), Lexchin noted that women were prescribed pharmaceuticals to cope with problems which stem from their subordinate role in society. Lexchin claims that drugs are prescribed by doctors to tranquillize women who are not complacent in traditional familial roles, when what is really needed is social change.

Women who use drugs have traditionally been perceived as more out of control (Inciardi, Lockwood, & Pottieger, 1993), deviant (Reed, 1987), and pathological than their male counterparts (Cuskey, 1982; Ettorre, 1992; Perry, 1979), even though men use more illicit drugs than women do (Addiction Research Foundation, 1994). Current and past research views women as more sexually promiscuous (see Inciardi et al., 1993; Reed, 1987; Stevenson, Lingley, Trasov, & Stansfield, 1956), more passive

(Perry, 1979), and morally weaker than men (Mondanaro, 1989). In addition, women who use drugs have been viewed as victims, both of drugs and of men who have led them astray (Maher, 1995). Traditional theory regarding women and drug use perceived women as passive and lacking agency (Henderson, 1993a; Maher, 1995).

The fact that there is little ethnographic[2] information about female illicit drug users is well documented (Addiction Research Foundation, 1994; Ettorre, 1992; Inciardi et al., 1993; Rosenbaum, 1981; Taylor, 1993). Historically, most research on illicit drugs has concentrated on male users (Addiction Research Foundation, 1994). The focus has been on 'the man about town,' rather than the mother at home with kids (see Biernacki, 1986; Hanson, Beschner, Walters, & Bovelle, 1985; Preble & Casey, 1969; Waldorf & Biernacki, 1979; Winick, 1962).

More recently, feminist qualitative research has begun to emerge that challenges the prevailing views about women who use illicit drugs (Colten, 1982; Dunlap & Johnson, 1996; Dunlap, Johnson, & Maher, 1997; Kearney, Murphy, & Rosenbaum, 1994; Knight et al., 1996; Morgan & Joe, 1997; Rosenbaum & Murphy, 1987). Several ethnographic sociological studies of women who use illicit narcotics exist, including Marsha Rosenbaum's (1981) study of female heroin users in San Francisco, California; Avril Taylor's (1993) study of female injectors in Glasgow, Scotland; Patricia Morgan and Karen Ann Joe's (1997) research on the illicit drug economy and methamphetamine use in three U.S. cities; and Lisa Maher's (1995) study of women in low-income minority neighbourhoods in Brooklyn, New York. Rosenbaum's (1981) and Taylor's (1993) studies are based on the sociological concept of 'career,' which was introduced by the Chicago School. Rosenbaum's focus is a career of narrowing options for women who use illicit drugs, and Taylor's is the strength and rational decision-making qualities of female drug users. In-depth interviews were conducted by both researchers, in addition to a fifteen-month period of participant observation by Taylor. Maher observed more than 200 women crack smokers during her three years of fieldwork in Brooklyn and gathered data from interviews with 45 women who lived on the street. Maher's ethnographic study successfully challenges conventional beliefs about women, crack cocaine, the drug trade, and the notion of agency. Morgan and Joe's study makes clear that 'most women who use and sell illicit drugs are not from minority disenfranchised populations living in large inner-city communities; most women who use and sell illicit drugs have not, and likely never will, engage in prostitution or felonious acts apart from illicit drug sale' (1997, p. 107). All four ethnographic studies focus on the user's perspective and contribute to a fuller understanding of the lives of women who use illicit drugs and they address the significance of the role of mothering to women who use illicit drugs.

Motherhood

Motherhood is central to the debates surrounding prenatal drug use and social service intervention. What constitutes mothering changes historically, and from culture to culture. Once thought to be a uniform, universal, instinctual response, mothering has been revealed by feminists to be a social construct, rather than a biological imperative (Glenn, 1994). Until recently, most Western research on mothering projected the concerns and experiences of white, upper-class women (Collins, 1994). Currently, many critical feminists have begun to examine not only the gender bias of research on mothering, but the race and class biases as well.

Adrienne Rich (1986) examines the concept of mothering as both experience and institution. She claims that motherhood can be a powerful and positive experience for women, but has been co-opted by complex interlocking forces – medicine, law, culture, and male expertise – which serve to control women's bodies and minds. Rich also discusses the successful struggles of women to resist outside definition and controls by patriarchal power.

The ideology of mothering[3] that pervades Western societies has made the actual unpaid work of mothering invisible. Since the Industrial Revolution, mothers have been romanticized as the givers of life and the caretakers of society's children, self-sacrificing and powerful in their maternal love. However, Kaplan (1994) notes how ideologies accommodate contradictory elements; thus women are also perceived as domineering, destructive, subordinate, and powerless against the forces of nature and instinct. Mothers are both feared and revered, and perceived as objects rather than subjects (Thurer, 1994).

During the Industrial Revolution the roles of women and children changed. Children were no longer economic contributors to the family. Rather, they were perceived as dependants in need of constant care and protection (Glenn, 1994; Mandell, 1995). Women were perceived as fit for the job of caring for the household and children because of their innate moral purity, self-sacrificing nature, and lack of intellect (Glenn, 1994). Child rearing and the production of children became a national and moral duty. However, in order to fulfil their duties properly, mothers needed to be instructed (Arnup, 1994; Davin, 1978). It was believed that mothers' ignorance led to social problems; therefore, classes were set up to educate mothers on proper hygiene and parenting skills. Rather than expanding social and medical services to ameliorate the myriad social problems related to the Industrial Revolution (such as high unemployment, lack of housing, poor working conditions, and unsanitary conditions), it was easier, cheaper, and consistent with ideological hegemony to blame mothers (Arnup, 1994; Davin, 1978).

Problems related to poverty were no longer defined as social; rather, public health and medical care were promoted as the cure for all family ills. With the advent of the public health and maternal health movements, motherhood has become a medicalized domain. Medical services that emphasized the surveillance of children, rather than care, and the professionalization of love, rather than the relationship between infant and mother, have become the norm during the twentieth century (Oakley, 1986).

The reality of mothering for most women, and especially for poor women and women of colour, has had little to do with virtue and caretaking of the future of society. Rather, it consists of long hours of unacknowledged and unpaid work and total responsibility for the care of dependants and household. Although some mothers are able to stay at home full-time with their children, most participate in outside employment (Segura, 1994).

Although the ideology of mothering that portrays women as giving, pure, and maternal permeates Western societies, women of colour and poor women are not enveloped by this mythology. Rather, they are perceived as incapable of nurturing and socializing children (Gupta, 1995), sexually promiscuous, having one baby after another (Solinger, 1994), and savage and animal-like (hooks, 1992). What is hidden by the ideology of mothering is the struggle by women of colour and poor women to have control over their own bodies, to have children, to keep the children they do have, and to protect their children from dominant ideologies that render their culture invisible (Collins, 1994). Slavery, the eugenics movement, forced sterilization and contraception, residential schools, child apprehension, and medical isolation of children diagnosed with neonatal abstinence syndrome (NAS) have served to prevent poor women and women of colour from having and keeping their own children.

Mothers, Illicit Drugs, and Parenting

In keeping with their suspected sexual immorality and their imagined compulsion and relentless drive to obtain their drugs through any means, women who use illicit drugs have been portrayed as deviating from traditional gender roles, especially with regards to motherhood. Often researchers and the media have constructed negative images of 'deviant mothers' who use illicit drugs (see Cain, 1994; Howard, Beckwith, Rodning, & Kropenske, 1989; Inciardi et al., 1993; Logli, 1990; Robertson, 1989; Shaw, 1985; Steinberg, 1994; Stone, Salerno, Green, & Zelson, 1971; Tait, 1996; Williams & Bruce, 1994). Mothers who use illicit drugs are portrayed as immature, out of control, deviant people; as 'unfit' mothers who pose a risk to their children (Taylor, 1993). Rosenbaum, Murphy, Irwin, and Watson (1990) note that the media have portrayed women who use illicit drugs as failing in their roles as mothers.

It is assumed that addicted parents fail to protect their children from harm, and the home environment is characterized as disruptive, chaotic (Howard et al., 1989, p. 8) and abusive (Chasnoff, 1988a; Jaudes, Ekwo, & Voorhis, 1995; Murphy et al., 1991; Peterson, Gable, & Saldana, 1996). Often writers state that parents (most often mothers) who use illicit drugs are incapable of caring for their children, and that their children are at risk for abuse (Dembo et al., 1990; Densen-Gerber & Rohrs, 1973; Howard et al., 1989; Jaudes et al., 1995; Kantor, 1978; Murphy et al., 1991; Weston, Ivins, Zuckerman, Jones, & Lopez, 1989). It is assumed that 'parents who are addicted to drugs have a primary commitment to chemicals, not to their children' (Howard et al., 1989, p. 8). Increasingly, illicit drug use during pregnancy is considered a 'direct form of child maltreatment' (Haskett, Miller, Whitworth, & Huffman, 1992, p. 451), and evidence of illicit drug use is often based on a positive urine toxicology report. Many U.S. states have enacted child abuse laws that extend to maternal drug use. Poor women and women of colour are subject to urine toxicology tests when they arrive at the hospital to give birth to their babies (Noble, 1997). Medical practitioners 'work hand and hand with child-welfare agents and the family and juvenile courts to define such women as child abusers' (Noble, 1997, p. 187).

Several studies imply that cocaine use impairs maternal behaviour (Johns, Noonan, Zimmerman, & Pedersen, 1994; Vernotica, Lisciotto, Rosenblatt, & Morrell, 1996). These studies – conducted on female rats injected with cocaine – claim that cocaine use may 'seriously compromise [mothers'] ability to nurture their infants' (Johns et al., 1994, p. 111). However, Alexander, Hadaway, and Coambs (1988) showed us that the utility of animal research is limited in the study of psychopathology. Their research clearly demonstrates that animals isolated in clinical settings differ from those that are socially housed. Research on animals given specific drugs in a clinical setting may not be applicable to humans in their natural environment (Morgan & Zimmer, 1997, pp. 149–50).

Researchers have speculated about the amount of discipline and punishment that exists in the families of origin of addicted persons. Some studies emphasize the lack of discipline in the families of origin (Hunt, 1974; Peterson, Gable, & Saldana, 1996; Robins, 1966; Seldin, 1972), while others note that mothers who use illicit drugs are too authoritarian (Wellisch & Steinberg, 1980) and overprotective (Bernardi, Jones, & Tennant, 1989).

In Chicago, Jaudes et al. (1995) reviewed hospital records from 1985 to 1990 for evidence of prenatal exposure to drugs through urine screening of newborns, together with information from the state central registry on allegations and investigations of child abuse. It was found that, over a period of five years, 513 infants had been exposed to drugs; allegations of abuse had been reported for 102 of the infants. Eighty per cent of the children were black. Neglect, rather than physical or sexual abuse, was the most common allegation, accounting for 72 per cent of cases among the 102 children. Physical injury was recorded for 15.7 and sexual abuse for 2.9 per cent of the children (Jaudes et al., 1995, p. 1068).

However, the authors state that 'no reliable information was available about the status of parental drug use at the time the child was abused' (Jaudes et al., 1995, p. 1069). In addition, the authors discovered that the risk of abuse increased along with higher levels of education of mothers, as did the rates of both planned abortions and miscarriage. The authors speculate that the increased risk may be explained by the mothers' frustration at having failed to live up to their potential – yet they did not interview the mothers.

Another study examined 'risk lists' obtained by court investigators in Boston. These lists were created to help court and social service workers evaluate degree and type of child abuse in families brought to court on care and protection petitions. The risk lists, court records, and documented and alleged substance abuse were examined for two years. Three-quarters of the children were from minority groups, poverty was pervasive, most of the families had single moms, and more than half were on welfare (Murphy et al., 1991, pp. 202, 208). The study used a control group of children whose parents were referred to the court but had no allegations of drug use against them (non-risk-rated sample). It was discovered that the rates of child abuse were similar in both groups, with neglect being the most common form (Murphy et al., 1991, p. 202). Alcohol was thought to be the most commonly used substance, followed by cocaine and heroin respectively (Murphy et al., 1991). The writers state that maternal substance abuse significantly increased the likelihood of parents being rated as 'high risk' to their children, of them rejecting court-ordered services, and of the permanent removal of children, despite both groups being referred to the court (Murphy et al., 1991, p. 208). In addition, alcohol-abusing parents were given more chances by social services and the court in relation to child-protection concerns than drug-abusing parents, even though alcohol-abusing parents had longer histories of children in need of protection, and more previous reports of mistreatment (Murphy et al., 1991, p. 208).

In conclusion, Murphy et al. (1991) stated that (alleged) substance abuse was only one of many problems the families in their sample faced. Others include lack of social support, parents having been abused in childhood, poverty, and lack of education. Murphy et al. (1991) suggest that these problems may be the true cause of child abuse or that substance abuse along with the factors listed above may have a 'co-occurring effect.' The authors warn that removing any one of these problems, including substance abuse, would not guarantee an abuse-free home situation.

Another study evaluating child-rearing attitudes and child-abuse 'potential' claimed that women who used drugs score higher than non-addicted women for child-abuse potential, although none of the women surveyed had abused her children; in fact, none of their babies was born yet (Williams-Petersen et al., 1994).

Many authors assume that the research on alcohol and families applies to illicit drug users, although there is no direct link. It has been suggested that alcoholism is linked to child abuse (Murphy et al., 1991; Steele, 1987). However, Steele (1987) claims that,

depending upon what particular population of abusers is studied or sampled, it can be shown with statistical significance that abusive, neglecting behavior can be precipitated or escalated by such things as poverty, bad housing, unemployment, marital strife, alcoholism, drug abuse, difficult pregnancies and deliveries, lack of education, lack of knowledge of child development, prematurity and illness of infants, deaths in the family, and a host of other things. (p. 82)

Steele points out that acknowledging social factors in situations of abuse does not answer the more basic question of why some people respond to stress with abusive behaviour while others do not (1987, p. 83). He concludes that abuse is generational and that abusers commonly have a history of neglect and abuse. However, not all adults abused as children go on to abuse their own children.

On reviewing all of the research in English on alcohol and child abuse published prior to 1981, Orme and Rimmer (1981) discovered that there was not enough empirical evidence to 'support an association between alcoholism and child abuse.' Many of the studies reviewed note that child abusers don't use any more alcohol than does the general population (Orme & Rimmer, 1981, p. 285). Orme and Rimmer conclude that writers have been mistaken in assuming that the correlation between alcoholism and child abuse is 'evidence of causation' (1981, p. 285).

Many studies suggest that people addicted to drugs have suffered trauma from their families during their formative years (Densen-Gerber & Rohrs, 1973; MacKinnon, 1991). It has been noted that certain groups of women who are addicted to drugs have experienced high rates of sexual and/or physical violence as children (Addiction Research Foundation, 1996; Mackinnon, 1991; Mondanaro, 1989; Pawl, 1992). However, the Addiction Research Foundation (1996) suggests that these findings may not be applicable to women in the general population. Because most research on sexual and/or physical abuse in the families of origin of illicit drug users has been conducted in treatment centres and prisons, the findings may not be applicable to the general population of illicit drug users. Russell and Wilsnack (1991) discovered that community studies outside of prison and drug treatment centres have shown lower levels of sexual abuse.

Maher's (1995) ethnographic research on women and crack cocaine challenges the uncritical acceptance of the idea that there is a causal relationship between early victimization and later drug use. Maher states that research which stresses the relationship between drug use and sexual abuse fails to examine other social factors, and drug use is reduced to a 'mere psychological effect' (1995, p. 5).

The only two ethnographic studies of women who use illicit drugs that preceded Maher's work, those of Rosenbaum (1981) and Taylor (1993), did not highlight sexual and/or physical abuse. Neither have numerous studies of both men and women (see Cheung, Erickson, & Landau, 1991; Erickson et al., 1987; Matthews, Dawes, Nadeau, Wong, & Alexander, 1995; Waldorf et al., 1991). Rather, these studies and others have begun to explore drug use as a social process which includes a wide range of motivations for continued use, both by women (Goode, 1994; Henderson, 1993a; Maher, 1995) and by men and women (Erickson et al., 1987; Matthews et al., 1995; Waldorf et al., 1991). These writers document that women use drugs for a wide range of reasons, including boredom, stress, anger management, reward, relaxation, and pleasure (Goode, 1994, p. 2).

Binion (1982) argues that family problems are just one of many factors which contribute to the development of addiction. Other contributing factors are interpersonal, social, and economic (Alexander, 1990; Binion, 1982).

The research on alcoholism, illicit drug use, and child abuse has been biased by an overrepresentation of families suffering from social and economic deprivation and of minority groups. Other flaws in the research include lack of empirical data, and failure to define abuse, alcoholism, and drug use. Bourne and Newberger state that our understanding of child abuse is 'at best intuitive and kind, at worst reflective and mean' (1979, p. 19). It appears that our understanding of drug use may be similar. The stigmatization and stereotyping of 'bad mothers' and 'loose women' continue to colour the discussion of maternal drug use.

Although illicit drug use is viewed as inconsistent with good mothering, many researchers have demonstrated that women who use illicit drugs can be adequate parents (Colten, 1980, 1982; Dreher, Nugent, & Hudgins, 1994; Hepburn, 1993a; Jackson & Berry, 1994; Kearney et al., 1994; Leeders, 1992; Lief, 1976; Sowder & Burt, 1980; Sterk-Elifson, 1996; Taylor, 1993; Zarin-Ackerman, 1976). Therefore, generalizations associating maternal drug use with child abuse must be made cautiously.

On reviewing the literature on mothers, illicit drugs, and parenting, it becomes apparent that mothers who use illicit drugs can be adequate parents. Both qualitative research with in-depth interviews (see Colten, 1982; Dreher et al., 1994; Jackson & Berry, 1994; Kearney et al., 1994; Leeders, 1992; Rosenbaum, 1981; Rosenbaum et al., 1990; Sterk-Elifson, 1996; Taylor, 1993), and research derived from programs designed to offer social, medical, and economic support to mothers who use illicit drugs and their children in a non-judgmental and non-punitive way (Hepburn, 1993a; Siney, 1994, 1995) confirm this.

Researchers have pointed out that the earliest ethnographic study on women and heroin (Rosenbaum, 1981) demonstrates that the 'interactions of drug use and motherhood were more fully apparent in ethnographic data than in findings from earlier surveys or closed-answer approaches' (Kearny et al., 1994, p. 352). Rosenbaum (1981) found that 'mothering' was the most important legitimate role of women who use heroin, and that their children were a stabilizing force in their lives. She also discovered that the women she interviewed saw themselves as primarily responsible for the caretaking of their children, and that the choice to stop using heroin was often influenced by the mother's concern for her children (1981, p. 104).

In 1980, Colten interviewed 170 women in treatment for heroin addiction, comparing them with a control group of 175 non-addicted women in the United States. Colten reported that the heroin-addicted mothers had just as much support and help from family and friends as did the non-addicted mothers (1982, p. 86). Like Rosenbaum (1981), Colten (1980, 1982) discovered that the 'mother' role was central to 'addicted' mothers, and that their relationships with their children did not differ from those of the non-addicted group. Their descriptions of their mothering experiences were similar to those of the non-addicted mothers; however, 'addicted' mothers used less physical forms of punishment than the non-addicted mothers and also reported using the tool of lecturing (verbal discipline) more often. Colten (1982) notes that these findings are particularly significant because women addicted to illicit drugs are often perceived as child abusers, although studies frequently fail to provide empirical data to support these claims.

Similarly, Sowder and Burt's (1980) study of 160 'addict' families and 160 non-addict families in five urban areas in the United States discovered that there was no difference between the two groups in terms of 'parents' childrearing practices and methods of discipline; parental expectations of their children; children's attitudes about school, and parents' perceptions of how well children were doing in school; [and] reports of abuse or neglect' (p. 19). Binion (1982) also notes that women who use heroin have more positive perceptions of their mothers than do non-addicted women.

Rosenbaum et al.'s (1990) study on women who use crack acknowledged that these mothers share the same parenting values as non-drug-using mothers. Ethnographic research on female narcotics users in Glasgow also demonstrates that these mothers have the same attitudes and hopes in mothering as the rest of society (Taylor, 1993). Kearney, Murphy, and Rosenbaum's qualitative study on mothering and crack cocaine explores how sixty-eight mothers in the San Francisco Bay area view mothering, including 'the strategies they used to manage mothering on cocaine, and the contextual influences on mothering outcomes' (1994, p. 351). Theidon (1995) examines how women who use illicit drugs utilize harm-reduction strategies to protect themselves and their families from their drug use and from violence in their lives. The above studies reveal that mothering is of central importance to the women interviewed, noting their distress when they are not able to carry out their maternal responsibilities.

Rather than suffering from physical abuse, children may be suffering because their mothers have limited financial and social resources and are subjected to 'rejection and disdain' (Colten, 1982, p. 88). Mothers who use illicit drugs are not offered much support; rather, their families are scrutinized by agencies and their children are taken away from them (Kearny et al., 1994, p. 360). Loss of custody of children was a reality for more than half of the mothers interviewed by Kearny, Murphy, and Rosenbaum (1994). Those who were able to place their children with family members retained a more favourable view of themselves as mothers (1994, p. 359). The mothers interviewed in this study described their successes and failures in relation to mothering, especially at times when socio-economic stress and other unexpected events prevented adequate mothering.

Leeders's (1992) two-year longitudinal study in the Netherlands (of thirty-five parents and their children who were 'hard' drug users, and thirty-one matched control foster families) demonstrates that a high percentage of the 'drug' families were doing well, with 'no significant correlations found between type or quantity of drug use, on the one hand, and various measures of parent–child interaction quality, on the other' (Leeders, 1992, p. 207).

Drawing from a study of seventy-eight African-American drug-dependent mothers in Los Angeles, Jackson and Berry describe how full-time mothering and 'responsibility for childcare is correlated with higher levels of maternal functioning' than part-time mothering (seeing the child between four times a week and once a month) (1994, p. 1532). It was discovered that the mothers who had full-time responsibility for their children displayed more positive attitudes than those who had only part-time responsibility (Jackson & Berry, 1994, p. 1528). Jackson and Berry (1994) conclude that keeping the family intact should be a primary goal, contrary to recent social welfare policy, which removes children from the home when maternal drug use is even suspected.

Women are given total responsibility, and held personally responsible, for the outcomes of their pregnancies and mothering, regardless of negative social and environmental factors. In the face of an ideology of mothering that ignores the social reality of women, and especially of poor women, women who use drugs are perceived as especially deviant. As previously noted it is often assumed that if they participate in one 'deviant' activity (illicit drug use) they will also participate in another (child abuse). Colten (1982) notes that addicted mothers had more concerns than did non-addicted mothers about their adequacy as mothers. She claims that these fears may be reinforced by societal responses to mothers who use illicit drugs. After all, much of the literature and the philosophy of drug treatment programs portrays mothers who use illicit drugs as bad parents. In contrast, men who use illicit drugs have not been subjected to a similar critique of their parenting skills.

Familial Ideology

The social control of women through familial ideology[4] and biological reproduction (sexuality, pregnancy, mothering) is significant in relation to women who use illicit drugs. The dominance of the nuclear family within legal and social policy tends to render all other family arrangements deviant in the eyes of family court and the criminal justice system. Early research by Carlen (1976), Daly (1987), and Eaton (1983, 1985) demonstrates that the courts give primacy to and uphold the dominance of the nuclear family, thereby exercising their 'overt' function of social control of women (Eaton, 1985). Outside of the criminal law, familial ideology also informs the decisions of social workers and medical professionals in the formation of policy and regulations.

Early research by Carlen (1976, 1983), Daly (1987), and Eaton (1983, 1985) emphasizes the impact of familial ideology on criminal and family court decisions. Carlen (1983) also pointed out how initial prison sentencing has immediate, devastating effects on women, as well as 'snowballing' effects. For example, when children are placed in care as a consequence of their mother's sentencing, that placement is often treated as significant evidence in determining future sentencing (Carlen, 1983). Furthermore, women sentenced to prison who had previously placed their children in care to protect them from battering husbands were not supported for these actions. Rather, their actions to protect their children were perceived by the courts as showing them to have failed as mothers (Carlen, 1983).

Gavigan claims that the dominant family form is basically 'defined and created by law' (1988, p. 289), and Masson's (1992) study of courtroom decisions in the Lower Mainland of British Columbia demonstrates that familial ideology is reflected in the sentencing of women in Canada. Masson (1992) interviewed nine Vancouver judges and examined 110 pre-sentence reports of women convicted of offences in Greater Vancouver, written between 1980 and 1991. On examination of the pre-sentence reports, Masson discovered that two of the most important variables affecting sentencing decisions were whether the defendants' children were in someone else's care, and the defendants' marital status (1992, pp.

iii, iv). Furthermore, the interviews with the judges demonstrated that they held ideas about proper female behaviour which were consistent with a patriarchal nuclear-family arrangement (Masson, 1992).

Assumptions about social reality often contain stereotypical ideals of feminism and family, and of the roles of both men and women in society (Chunn & Gavigan, 1991; Daly, 1989; Gavigan, 1993; Edwards, 1981; MacKinnon, 1987). These assumptions or ideologies are internalized by both lawmakers and enforcers, influencing and contributing '*indirectly* to the reproduction of class, gender, and racial/ethnic inequalities' (Chunn & Gavigan, 1991, p. 302). Familial ideology explains disparities in sentencing for similar offences; female offenders who have 'normal families' and assume appropriate gender roles often receive more lenient sentencing (Daly, 1989; Eaton, 1986; Masson, 1992; Simpson, 1989). Similar disparities can be witnessed in the medical (Gallagher, 1987) and social service professions (Chunn, 1995; Maher, 1992; Maier, 1992). Thus, sentencing decisions are often 'family based rather than individual based' (Daly, 1989, p. 11).

The families of origin of illicit drug users have been portrayed as pathological and unorganized (Binion, 1982, p. 44). However, the availability of family and extended family is explored in Dunlap and Johnson's (1996) case study of the development of a female crack-seller in the United States. They contend that the availability of family resources greatly influences the extent to which female illicit drug users can maintain a '"normal identity" and a "stake in conventional life"' (Dunlap & Johnson, 1996, p. 175). Thus, the importance of extended family should be primary in any discussion of women who use illicit drugs.

The social control of women in Western societies has been carried out primarily through the regulation of family norms, mothering, sexuality, and reproduction. All women are subject to these controls. But women who use illicit drugs have become the battlefield for the increased surveillance, control, and punishment of all women who do not conform to dominant ideologies of mothering.

Reproductive Autonomy

Feminists have argued that women are subjected to specific forms of social control because of their capacity to become pregnant. Traditionally, pregnancy was discussed as an individual event. However, recent discourse has broadened our concept of reproduction and the social constraints surrounding it. Maternal drug use has recently become controversial. Mothers have been detained, arrested, and subjected to medical interventions as a result of their status as suspected illicit drug users.

Historically, the realm of reproduction was woman-centred. Female healers and midwives attended to women's reproductive needs (Ehrenreich & English, 1973). Midwifery was a holistic practice that supported the mother and celebrated birth (Martin, 1992). Pregnancy and birth were not 'synonymous with illness' (Burtch, 1994, p. 55). Midwives have traditionally been the 'guardians of normal birth.'

During the late nineteenth and early twentieth centuries, the newly established medical profession strengthened its fragile position by defining pregnancy and birth and appropriating them from non-professional women (mothers, aunts, etc.) who helped deliver children, traditional midwives, and healers (Ehrenreich & English, 1973; Oakley, 1984). Legislation was passed in most of Canada during the twentieth century that rendered the practice of midwifery illegal. Pregnancy and birth were now defined in Canada as medical events that required doctors, nurses, and specialized technology (Burtch, 1994). Lobbying efforts, medical 'science,' and the policing of rebellious doctors and deviant or 'immoral women' led to the medical profession's acquisition of control over many aspects of women's lives (McLaren, 1978).

Women were considered ignorant in the areas of pregnancy, childbirth, and childcare. This justified the surveillance and control of these areas by the newly established medical profession (Arnup, 1994; Oakley, 1984). The emergence of antenatal care in the early twentieth century shaped women's experience of pregnancy, birth, and mothering (Arnup, 1994; Oakley, 1984).

The obstetrical pursuit of more and more knowledge about the foetus *in utero* is an important aspect of the medical profession's claim to legitimacy. New antenatal interventions have allowed the obstetrical community to acquire information about the foetus without using the mother as intermediary (Oakley, 1984). The mystification of pregnancy by the male-dominated medical profession and the emergence of reproductive technology have limited women's knowledge of their bodies (Smart & Smart, 1978). Mothers lack information about their pregnancies, and the period before birth has been opened to medical scrutiny and expertise.

The history of the medical treatment of women in Canada emphasizes the continuing struggle by women to define their own experience of birth, menopause, and menstruation, and to rebel against the medical profession's moral stance on their proper role in the family and in society (Mitchinson, 1991).

Foetal Rights

Prior to the nineteenth century, women in Canada were not restricted from obtaining birth control or abortion before quickening (Brodie, Gavigan, & Jenson, 1992; McLaren, 1990). Even though the use of birth control and abortion were criminalized in the nineteenth century, Canadian women continued to obtain birth control and abortions illegally. The use of birth control and abortion were legalized in Canada in 1969; however, at that time abortion was not a woman's right. Rather, it became a medical matter, where therapeutic abortion committees decided which women were eligible (Brodie et al., 1992). Currently, therapeutic abortion committees no longer exist in Canada, and women have improved access to abortion.

Since the advent of legal abortion in Canada, the foetal rights movement has gained considerable leverage. The representation of the foetus as a person with sovereign rights has led to a questioning and erosion of women's rights, and the foetus and the mother are viewed as adversaries. Brodie et al. note that 'there is an obvious political imperative to protect the foetus against the destructive impulses of the pregnant woman' (1992, p. 83).

However, the characteristics that compel us to recognize 'personhood' do not appear until long after birth. 'Foetal personhood' is a *decision*, not a medical or legal discovery (Callahan & Knight, 1992, p. 129). The medical model of birth and of the female body has led to the perception of the uterus as a machine, the woman as a labourer, and the baby as the product. Doctors are concerned with foetal outcome, not with the mother and the delivery (Martin, 1987, p. 64). New technologies facilitating contact with the foetus have led to an extension of the moment of 'personhood' (Oakley, 1984). Legal and medical discourses in relation to the foetus legitimize their hidden assumptions about women and mothering through science and its 'claim to truth' (Fitzgerald, 1993, p. 3). And 'the boundary between what constitutes the "good" mother and the "bad" mother has become clearly delineated in terms of a medical-scientific definition' (p. 18).

As well, the image of the foetus as separate from the mother, documented in medical textbooks, has emerged as a visual representation of life and death. Anti-abortionists were quick to recognize the potential of the visual representation of the foetus (Petchesky, 1990). Consequently, foetal personhood has become a symbol for the anti-choice movements in Canada and the United States (Brodie et al., 1992; Fitzgerald, 1993; Petchesky, 1990).

The impact of foetal rights is highlighted in Kolder, Gallagher, and Parsons's (1987) documentation of court-ordered obstetrical interventions in the United States. They discovered that 81 per cent of court-ordered interventions directed at pregnant women were for black, Asian, or Hispanic women; 44 per cent were unmarried; and none was a private patient (1987, p. 1192). The symbolic importance of the foetus, and court-ordered caesareans, conveys important legal and moral messages to women concerning their status in society. Medical technology and prenatal medical interventions have advanced foetal rights, and 'spurred a resurgence of powerful, largely unacknowledged social attitudes in which pregnant women are viewed and treated as vessels' (Gallagher, 1989, p. 188).

The controversy emerging over court-ordered interventions and foetal rights is also noted by Maier (1992) in her case study of 'Baby R' in Vancouver, B.C. Maier examined court-ordered caesareans and developed the term 'reproductive violation,' which includes forcible confinement and reproductive violence (1992, p. 84). The criminalization and imprisonment of pregnant women in the United States who use illicit drugs (in order to protect the foetus from exposure to maternal drug use) falls under Maier's category of reproductive violation.

According to Shaw (1985), if 'the mother decides to carry a foetus to term, she incurs a conditional prospective liability toward her foetus that ripens at live birth' (1985, p. 314) and she claims that the child should be able to sue the mother for 'wrongful prenatal care.' Robertson (1989) contends that incarcerating pregnant women is preferable to incarcerating women after birth, for foetal harm may be avoided. Furthermore, he argues that incarceration will be cheaper in the long run, for it will lower the cost of caring for the disabled children of drug addicts (Robertson, 1989). Logli (1990) agrees that 'once a pregnant woman has abandoned her right to abort and has decided to carry the foetus to term, society can well impose a duty on the mother to insure that the foetus is born as healthy as possible' (1990, p. 26).

In *Roe v. Wade* (1973), the U.S. Supreme Court noted that the state's interest became compelling when the foetus became viable, or able to live outside the mother's body. In the landmark decision in *Morgentaler v. The Queen* (1988), it became clear that all of the Canadian Supreme Court justices involved were committed to 'state interest in the foetus ... if not full legal personality' (Brodie et al., 1992, p. 127). Canadian Justice Wilson states that the state may be compelled to have an interest in the foetus, depending on its gestational age. The Law Reform Commission of Canada (1989) states that women have a moral obligation to their foetus to avoid harm, and the 'foetus merits at least some protection, not necessarily of the same order as that accorded to those already born, but of a kind increasing as it develops' (p. 7).

Foetal rights legislation raises the question of foetal harm and protection. As previously mentioned, often the foetus and the mother are viewed as adversaries. With the advancement of reproductive technology, the moment of foetal viability is continually extended, and women's rights diminish accordingly. The representation of the foetus as a person with sovereign rights has led to a questioning and erosion of women's rights. The arguments for legal personhood of the foetus have contributed to expanding state control of all pregnant women and of birthing choices (Gallagher, 1989).

Proposals to compel pregnant women to accept medical treatment and criminal and civil liability impose 'new and unique legal duties on pregnant women' (Martin & Coleman, 1995, p. 990). However, several authors claim that foetal rights have not been judicially recognized in Canada (Flagler, Baylis, & Rodgers, 1997; Martin & Coleman, 1995). It has been pointed out that the Supreme Court, in *Brooks v. Canada Safeway Ltd.*, 'established that discrimination on the basis of pregnancy is discrimination on the basis of sex, even though only women have the capacity to become pregnant' (Martin & Coleman, 1995, p. 984). Martin and Coleman (1995) note that the 1993 Royal Commission on New Reproductive Technologies in Canada expressed concern about judicial intervention in pregnancy on the grounds that such intervention would not reflect women's *Charter* rights.[5] The commission recommended:

273. Judicial intervention in pregnancy and birth not be permissible. Specifically, the Commission recommends that:

a. medical treatment never be imposed upon a pregnant woman against her wishes;

b. the criminal law, or any other law, never be used to confine or imprison a pregnant woman in the interest of her foetus;

c. the conduct of a pregnant woman in relation to her foetus not be criminalized;

d. child welfare or other legislation never be used to control a woman's behaviour during pregnancy or birth; and

e. civil liability never be imposed upon a woman for harm done to her foetus during pregnancy.

274. Unwanted medical treatment and other interferences, or threatened interferences, with the physical autonomy of pregnant women be recognized explicitly under the *Criminal Code* as criminal assault. (Royal Commission on New Reproductive Technologies, 1993, p. 964).

It is often assumed that 'protective' foetal legislation will enhance the health of the developing foetus and the pregnant mother. However, Smart notes that health promotion is not 'intrinsically good.' Rather, it can have very serious ramifications for women and infants, especially when women's bodies are perceived as 'central to the health of others' (1989, p. 99). Medical concern with foetal health and healthy pregnancies, which is constructed as a desirable goal, can be 'transposed into oppressive forms of legislation which assume the terminology of benevolence and public health' (Smart, 1989, p. 98). The focus on foetal health has led to discriminatory practices against all women, and especially women who use illicit drugs. Non-drug-using women in North America have been subject to court-ordered obstetrical interventions, urine testing for drug use, and instructions by health professionals that have little to do with the needs of the mother. Seeing women's bodies as 'central to the health of others' can lead to discriminatory practices against women (Smart, 1989, p. 98).

A recent case in Winnipeg, Manitoba, clearly illuminates how Canadian women's Charter rights can be infringed upon when maternal drug use is viewed as neglect and abuse, and women's bodies are viewed as central to the health of others. In 1996, Winnipeg Child and Family Services brought forward an application to have the court force a young pregnant women who was alleged to be addicted to solvents to enter drug treatment. The case received national attention when Mr Justice Perry Schulman of the Manitoba Court of Queen's Bench ordered that the woman be confined to a drug treatment centre until her baby was born. The media portrayed this woman as already having two older children who suffered from 'brain damage' due to her solvent use. It is assumed that there is a link between solvent use and foetal damage during pregnancy. In fact, 'a definable foetal solvent syndrome (FSS) has not yet been demonstrated' (Addiction Research Foundation, 1997, p. 2).

Medrano's (1996) critical review of forty-two studies on foetal solvent syndrome (FSS), or toluene embryopathy, concludes that all of the studies were descriptive cases of voluntary and involuntary maternal exposure. Although many of the studies reported congenital defects and spontaneous abortions, the shortcomings of the methods employed and the failure to consider the use of either alcohol or other drugs, or the length of exposure, limited their usefulness. Medrano states that 'a discrete FSS has not been demonstrated at this time' (1996, p. 73).

On appeal, the Manitoba Court of Appeal unanimously declared that child welfare authorities cannot force pregnant women into drug treatment and that the rights of the mother take precedence because the foetus is not a person in law (Mitchell, 1996). Their decision affirmed that a pregnant woman cannot be forced to undergo drug treatment and medical treatment to protect the foetus (Mitchell, 1996). The young women in question subsequently gave birth to a healthy infant. On appeal, the Supreme Court of Canada agreed to hear the case. On 31 October 1997, the Supreme Court of Canada held that the courts cannot force pregnant women into drug treatment for the purpose of protecting the unborn child. In the decision, the Court upheld that 'the law of Canada does not recognize the unborn child as a legal person possessing rights' (*Winnipeg Child and Family Services [Northwest Area] v. G. [D.F.]*, 1997).

The focus on deviant pregnant women distracts society from addressing such issues as racial and class bias, 'foetal protection' policies, the poor maternal health and infant mortality rates in the United States (which are the highest among all Western nations), and the lack of services and resources 'that enable women to have healthy babies' (Chavkin, 1992, p. 200). Nsiah-Jefferson (1989) argues that poor women and women of colour have always been held personally responsible for poor reproductive outcomes. Furthermore, nine months of antenatal care during pregnancy 'cannot offset years of poor health' (Mitchinson, 1988, p. 259).

The role of the medical profession as an agent of social control 'and arbiter of reproductive behavior' (Stephenson & Wagner, 1993, p. 174) has been challenged by critical and feminist social researchers. Historically, and in contemporary society, pregnant women have been instructed on how to behave and restricted from engaging in certain activities. Women have been told to avoid exercise, or to be sure to exercise daily. They've been instructed to have an alcoholic beverage before bedtime to induce sleep (in the 1950s), or to abstain from alcohol. They've been ordered to eat well, to reduce weight, to take vitamins, to take drugs prescribed by their doctors (including Thalidomide, phenobarbital, and amphetamines). Still, we rarely perceive doctors as hazardous to pregnancy. Rather, the mother is perceived as a source of harm

(Rothman, 1989). Pregnant women are presented with obligations for every waking moment of their day (King, 1989), and these obligations rarely reflect their desires.

According to Faith, 'medicine provides the scientific framework within which female subordination is ideologically justified and law supplies the mechanism' (1993, p. 45). For women who use illicit drugs in North America, the arm of the law 'retains its "old" power ... whilst exercising new contrivances of power in the form of surveillance and modes of discipline' (Smart, 1989, p. 17). These 'contrivances' include the medical and social services professions. Although women who are suspected of illicit drug use suffer from these new controls, all women, to some extent, have been subject to social service, legal, and medical regulation in Western societies since the late 1800s (Oakley, 1984).

Feminists conclude that the criminalization of pregnancy (Callahan & Knight, 1992; Chavkin, 1992; Humphries et al., 1992; Maher, 1992; Mariner, Glantz, & Annas, 1990) and emerging foetal rights have culminated in a situation where the well-being and security of women's bodies are legally and physically challenged (Gallagher, 1987, 1989; Martin, 1987; Oakley, 1984; Petchesky 1990).

In addition, Oakley (1984) states that motherhood has been co-opted by the scientism of medicine. Women who use illicit drugs are often challenged by the legal, medical, and social service professions once their children are born, for it is thought that illicit drug use equals poor parenting, which places children at risk.

Maternal Drug Use

The majority of social science research concerning maternal drug use has emerged from the United States, where legal sanctions pertaining to prenatal exposure to illicit drugs have been put in place. Women who use illicit drugs have recently been subject to legal, welfare, and medical regulation. Medical regulation of illicit drug users focusing on maternal heroin use emerged in the 1960s. Regulation focusing on cocaine use emerged in the 1980s. Social welfare professionals began to view maternal drug use as a social problem in the mid-1980s.

In the United States, legal sanctions against maternal drug use have been initiated by thirty states since the mid-1980s (Center for Reproductive Law & Policy, 1996). Also in the United States, between 1985 and 1995 an estimated 200 women have been arrested on criminal charges stemming from their behaviour during pregnancy; most of the prosecutions are based on 'allegations' of illicit drug use during pregnancy (Center for Reproductive Law & Policy, 1996). Prosecutors have used legal statutes intended for other purposes and extended them to encompass pregnant women (Paltrow, 1992). Many of these cases involve doctors who contacted legal authorities about the mothers' suspected illicit drug use (Stephenson & Wagner, 1993).

Mothers have been arrested for child abuse and neglect, child endangerment, drug possession, assault with a deadly weapon, manslaughter, homicide, and trafficking to the foetus *in utero*. All these charges pertain to allegations of taking drugs while pregnant. This raises the question of whether a 'foetus' is protected by law prior to birth. In the cases where race was identified, 70 per cent of the women charged between 1985 and 1992 were women of colour (Paltrow, 1992).

Legal attention focuses on lifestyle and assumed increase in female use of illicit drugs. Bloom, Chesney-Lind & Owen (1994) describe the increase in the number of drug-using women imprisoned in the United States, where one out of three women is serving time for drug offences (an increase from one in ten in 1979). Over a third of these women are serving time for 'possession' (Bloom et al., 1994, p. 1).

Women who use illicit drugs often lose custody of their infants at birth or later, due to social service intervention. In Canada, mothers who use illicit drugs are perceived as placing their children at risk. Feminists have introduced the term 'the criminalization of pregnancy' to describe legal sanctions against pregnant women in Western society. Discourse centres on *suspected* maternal harm to the foetus and *conjectured* prenatal harm as child abuse. In North America, laws pertaining to 'legal persons' have been applied to the foetus, and mothers have been arrested, incarcerated, and subjected to medical and surgical interventions in order to prevent 'foetal harm' (Kolder et al., 1987). In Canada, First Nations women, poor women, and single mothers appear to be overrepresented in terms of arrests, child apprehensions, and medical interventions (Chunn & Gavigan, 1991; LaPrairie, 1987; McLaren, 1990; Monture, 1989).

Most feminist research concerning maternal drug use has failed to examine the social construction of 'good' and 'bad' drugs, the consequent negative effects of the Controlled Drugs and Substances Act, and the social construction of neonatal abstinence syndrome (NAS). Most feminist and non-feminist research on maternal drug use overlooks how punitive legal, medical, and social service policy stems from the criminalization of specific drugs as well as from social attitudes regarding women, reproduction, and mothering. There has been little critique by either feminists or non-feminists concerning the authenticity of NAS as a medical diagnosis and the consequent medical care of infants labelled with NAS. However, assumptions regarding the harm of illicit drugs to foetal health inform medical, social service, and legal policy.

Neonatal Abstinence Syndrome (NAS)

It is difficult to acquire accurate information concerning prenatal exposure to drugs, as many authors tend to make statements which have very little scientific validity (Koren, 1997; Mayes, Granger, Bornstein, & Zuckerman, 1992). Since the 1950s, it has been evident that the medical profession is sceptical of information obtained from illicit drug users in relation to the quality and quantity of their drug use. Women were especially suspect when pregnant, and since the early 1960s doctors have discussed the denial and manipulation displayed by pregnant women who used illicit drugs.

It is argued that infants need to be identified early so that protection and medical attention can be available to them (Peak & Papa, 1993; Robin-Vergeer, 1990). Ultrasound and electronic monitoring are recommended for validating the accuracy of mothers' observations of foetal activity (Robins & Mills, 1993, p. 26). Drug screening and increased surveillance of all newborns are advocated when there is a history of maternal drug use, and meconium (the first intestinal discharges of the newborn) is found in the amniotic fluid. As well, meconium testing and hair analysis are used in some hospitals. Many researchers discuss how promising these new techniques for assessment of prenatal drug exposure are (Albersheim, 1994; Robins & Mills, 1993), without fully addressing the ethics of subjecting mothers and infants to medical testing with or without consent.

In utero drug exposure is usually determined through drug testing (urine analysis) of mothers during delivery. Often identification of maternal drug use is based on *suspected* illicit drug use because urine analysis, the primary form of drug testing, is unreliable. Drug testing can only tell what drugs were used within the previous twenty-four to seventy-two hours (Humphries et al., 1992). Drug testing cannot distinguish the dependent, occasional, or first-time user, and, as Humphries et al. (1992) discuss, there is a race and class bias associated with drug testing in the United States. Most important, drug testing cannot determine whether an infant will be adversely affected by its mother's drug use.

The long- and short-term affects of maternal use of narcotics (opium

derivatives) are somewhat controversial. Since the advent of criminalization of narcotics in Canada and most Western countries, health problems
associated with narcotics are difficult to distinguish from health problems
related to the illicit status of the drug and to the users' socio-economic
environment.

Early medical research on maternal narcotic use noted that heroin use
caused intrauterine growth retardation, microcephaly (small head circumference), stress (Naeye, Branc, Leblanc, & Khatamee, 1973), and
spontaneous abortion (Rementeria & Nunag, 1973). In 1979, Finnegan
(1979) reported and diagnosed neonatal abstinence syndrome (NAS),
establishing guidelines for care. Higher rates for sudden infant death syndrome were attributed to maternal heroin use (a five- to tenfold increase)
(Chasnoff, 1988b). In addition, low birth weight and length, and withdrawal symptoms, have most often been attributed to prenatal exposure
to narcotics. More recently, withdrawal (Hepburn, 1993a, 1993b), low
birthweight associated with cigarette smoking, and pre-term delivery
(Siney, 1994; Siney, Kidd, Waldinshaw, Morrison, & Manasse, 1995) appear to be the most serious problems associated with maternal drug
use.

Prior to 1980, studies of maternal drug use concentrated on heroin and
methadone. Infants experiencing withdrawal were said to experience
problems ranging from flu-like symptoms and tremors to dehydration
and, possibly, death. Early medical studies cited infant withdrawal as a
specific effect of maternal narcotic use and discussed the suffering infants
experienced as a result of their mother's illicit drug use. Stern states that
all children of mothers who use heroin will be born 'addicted and with
withdrawal symptoms' (1966, p. 255). Physicians became advocates for
'prevention of unnecessary suffering of infants unable to express their
agony while going through this phase' (Fricker & Segal, 1978, p. 366).
Currently, many doctors believe that saving these infants takes precedence over 'abstract concepts of rights and autonomy' for women (Steinberg, 1994, p. 17).

However, the only specific effect of maternal narcotic use is infant withdrawal, and not all infants exposed prenatally to narcotics experience
symptoms of withdrawal. Any discussion of infant withdrawal is incomplete and biased if it does not emphasize the fact that withdrawal is transitory and is not predictable (as not all infants exhibit withdrawal
symptoms). The onset and duration of withdrawal vary even when the
same drug is being studied in different infants. At the Women's Reproductive Health Service in Glasgow, of 200 babies born to women who

used drugs during pregnancy only 7 per cent required treatment for withdrawal symptoms, and fewer still were admitted to a special care nursery (Hepburn, 1993b, p. 54). The Liaison Antenatal Drug Service in South London noted that none of the infants seen was admitted to a special care unit after birth in the first year the service was established. The South London program, which saw only thirty-five mothers during that year, appears to have reduced withdrawal symptoms in their infants (Latchem, 1994, p. 486). In contrast, the number of infants requiring treatment for withdrawal in the United States and Canada has been cited as ranging from 60 to 95 per cent of the total number of infants prenatally exposed to drugs. The question is, why is there such a large variance between percentages in the U.K. and North American studies? In Glasgow, Hepburn has discovered that poor pregnancy outcomes 'may be due not so much to the drugs as to the underlying socioeconomic deprivation or the effects of drug use on lifestyle' (1993b, p. 54).

Cocaine-related difficulties during pregnancy were first reported by Acker, Sachs, and Tracey in 1983. An increase in placental abruption (Acker et al., 1983) and neurobehavioural abnormalities in infants (Chasnoff, Burns, Schnoll, & Burns, 1985) were attributed to maternal cocaine use. As well, an increase in prenatal morbidity and sudden infant death syndrome were noted (Chasnoff, 1988b). The most common effects noted in medical research include intense vasoconstriction (reduced oxygen supply due to blood vessel constriction), which contributes to low birth weight, small head circumference, and increased risk of premature birth. Teratogenic effects, birth anomalies, and developmental and behavioural problems have also been cited. Finally, infants have been found to be irritable and difficult to care for, and failure to attach or bond has been observed.

Subsequent research has challenged many early claims of life-threatening problems in infants prenatally exposed to cocaine (see Chasnoff, Griffith, Freier, & Murray, 1992; Frank & Zuckerman, 1993; Greider, 1995; Hawley & Disney, 1992; Institute for the Study of Drug Dependence [ISDD], 1992; Lindenberg et al., 1991; Matthews, 1993; Mayes et al., 1992; Morgan & Zimmer, 1997; Myers, Olson, & Kaltenbach, 1992; Robins & Mills, 1993). For example, the incidence of placental abruption is controversial (Lindenberg, Alexander, Gendrop, Nencioli, & Williams, 1991; Robins & Mills, 1993). Hepburn (1993a) noted that higher incidences of placental abruption did not occur in her Glasgow study, nor did other obstetric complications often cited in relation to prenatal drug use.

Furthermore, the association between sudden infant death syndrome

(SIDS) and maternal cocaine use is not firmly established (Hepburn, 1993a; Humphries, 1993; Koren, 1997; Mayes et al., 1992). Brown and Zuckerman state that recent studies show no increased risk or 'slightly elevated risk,' which may be associated with socio-economic deprivation (1991, p. 563). Hepburn (1993a) has not found major increases in perinatal morbidity as a result of maternal drug use, including cocaine use.

Infants exposed to cocaine prenatally are said to have low birth weight and small head circumference. However, Brown and Zuckerman note that 'this effect on growth is probably compounded by maternal undernutrition and poly-drug abuse' (1991, p. 561), which could include the use of cigarettes and alcohol (Robins & Mills, 1993). Importantly, the large majority of infants exposed to cocaine prenatally are not low birth weight (Robins & Mills, 1993; Myers, Olson, & Kaltenbach, 1992). Nulman et al.'s (1994) study of twenty-three cocaine-exposed infants and their adopted mothers, and twenty-three matched control children not exposed to cocaine and their adopted mothers, suggests that prematurity and smaller head circumference may be attributable to intrauterine cause rather than environmental factors. However, further research is needed in order to determine the validity of their claims, as their sample was small and they excluded factors related to the mother's age and the adoption process, which may be significant.

Prematurity is associated with low birth weight, but the majority of infants exposed prenatally to cocaine are not premature (Myers et al., 1992). As well, infants with low birth weight may be tested for maternal drug use more often than infants born within the range of normal birth weight, which would bias findings (Robins & Mills, 1993). Brown and Zuckerman (1991) also note that mothers who tested negative for urine toxicology at the time of birth, but reported having used cocaine during their pregnancies, did not give birth to infants with low birth weight. Shorter body length of infants exposed prenatally to cocaine is attributed to their mothers' drug use, but may actually be caused by maternal undernutrition (Brown & Zuckerman, 1991).

While it is still controversial whether infants exposed to cocaine may experience withdrawal, certainly the specific effects noted in infants experiencing opiate withdrawal are not evident (Hepburn, 1993b; Myers et al., 1992; Morgan & Zimmer, 1997; Morrison & Siney, 1996). Nor is there evidence to support long-term sequelae in infants experiencing withdrawal symptoms due to maternal drug use (Hepburn, 1993a). Many studies detect no differences between infants exposed to cocaine prenatally and non-exposed infants. However, these studies have not been readily available in professional journals. Koren, Graham, Shear, and Ein-arson (1989) discovered that studies which found no difference in cocaine-exposed infants and non-exposed infants were rejected for pre-sentation at scientific meetings and conferences, and by journals, more often than were studies which supported the incidence of adverse effects in infants prenatally exposed to cocaine. This practice ignores the supe-rior methodology used in the studies demonstrating no difference between the two groups of infants. Evidently, the ideology surrounding NAS and illicit drug use is so entrenched that conflicting empirical evi-dence is disregarded by the scientific community.

Behavioural problems are often associated with children prenatally exposed to cocaine. However, critics state that it is not yet possible to determine whether behavioural problems are caused by maternal drug use (Hepburn, 1993b; Mayes et al., 1992), as studies do not take into account exposure to other drugs, genetic liabilities, and prenatal liabili-ties (Robins & Mills, 1993, p. 18). Many of the behaviours that researchers describe in infants exposed to maternal drug use are identical to behav-iours found in 'unusually small babies' (Robins & Mills,1993, p. 18). Infants exposed to cocaine prenatally are often said to be recognizable by their behavioural differences and their 'unreachableness' in interper-sonal relationships. But Robins and Mills note that children exposed to drugs are no different from other children from economic and socially deprived backgrounds (1993, p. 29). And Hawley and Disney (1992) point out that children who remained with their biological mothers were securely attached. There is no information about children exposed pre-natally to cocaine whose families were not identified through welfare agencies (Hawley & Disney, 1992), and those children outside of the wel-fare system may have no identifiable problems.

Infants who have been exposed prenatally to cocaine have been said to be permanently affected by their mothers' drug use. But 'predictions of an adverse developmental outcome for these children are being made despite a lack of supportive scientific evidence,' state Mayes et al. (1992, p. 406). Maternal cocaine use is unlikely to be the cause of so many unsubstantiated effects on infant health. Myers et al. (1992) conclude that 'the simple truth at this point is that we do not yet know what the effects are of prenatal cocaine exposure' (1992, p. 1). There is no known syndrome related to prenatal exposure to cocaine that produces a set of recognizable physiological and mental deficiencies. According to Myers et al., there are '*no* published studies of middle- and upper-class cocaine-using mothers and their infants. Rather, low-income women make up the study populations. This means that the conditions of poverty get mixed up with effects of cocaine exposure' (1992, p. 4).

Although adverse effects of prenatal cocaine exposure are presented in the literature, the majority of infants exposed to cocaine prenatally are not impaired (Hawley & Disney, 1992). Many of the problems associated with maternal drug use have nothing to do with a specific drug's pharmacological action, but are related 'to the way they are used, the illegality of their use and other adverse factors predisposing to or resulting from drug use' (Hepburn, 1993a, p. 54). Cocaine is not the monster claimed by the press and the majority of scientific studies. It is one variable among many that influence maternal outcomes. So far it has been impossible to isolate maternal cocaine use from other variables that affect pregnancy outcomes, such as poverty (Morgan & Zimmer, 1997; Myers et al., 1992).

Although cigarettes are thought to cause the same kinds of prenatal effects as cocaine and opiates, such as low birth weight, tobacco is rarely included in maternal drug studies that determine foetal harm (see Chasnoff, Harvey, Landress, & Barrett, 1990). As well, there seems to be more credible evidence that prenatal exposure to alcohol may contribute to foetal alcohol syndrome (FAS), though few maternal drug studies have included alcohol as a variable. However, Koren notes that 'only chronic, heavy drinking has been associated with foetal anomalies' (1997, p. 54). Unlike alcohol use, prenatal exposure to cocaine and narcotics has not yet been empirically linked to a 'syndrome.' Maternal drug research clearly demonstrates that alcohol and tobacco *use* are common among mothers who do not use illicit drugs (Higgins, Moxley, Pencharz, Mikolainis, & Dubois, 1989), and mothers who are illicit drug users (Chasnoff, 1989; Chasnoff et al., 1990; Graham & Koren, 1991; Siney, 1995). Often more than 80 per cent of pregnant women who use illicit drugs test positive for tobacco in research studies (Boer & Kreyenbroek, 1989; Fulroth, Phillips, & Durand, 1989; Mastrogiannis, Decavalas, Verma, & Tejani, 1990). In 1994, 66.7 per cent of women (aged fifteen and older) in Canada reported that they were current alcohol drinkers, and 25.6 per cent stated that they currently smoked tobacco (McKenzie, Williams, & Single, 1997, p. 33,75). It is also documented that tobacco smokers drink more alcohol than do non-smokers (McKenzie et al., 1997). But studies in the past relating smoking to low birth weight failed to reveal how tobacco use is associated with heavy alcohol use (Chasnoff, 1988a, 1988b). Siney et al. (1995) state that a reduction of cigarette smoking is the overall aim of their maternity services in Liverpool.

Rarely do social science, medical, and legal articles emphasize the low percentage of illicit drug use demonstrated in urine toxicology studies related to maternal drug use. Rather, the total results for all maternal drug use (licit and illicit) are advanced to support increased regulation and monitoring of pregnant women (see Chasnoff et al. 1990; Kaye, Elkind, Goldberg, & Tytun, 1989; Peak & Papa, 1993; Robins & Mills, 1993). Consequently, the negative ideology concerning illicit drug use remains intact. As well, though some research challenges what urine toxicology screening data for illicit drugs tell us, it fails to analyse the significant use of legal drugs and the use of marijuana (our most benign drug) in relation to other illicit drugs. A growing number of feminist writers have begun to examine the lack of analysis regarding licit drugs in research models (see Blume, 1992; Gieringer, 1990; Humphries et al., 1992; Merlo, 1993; Siney, 1995; Siney et al., 1995).

Since illicit drug use is only one variable of many that may affect pregnancy, cigarette smoking, alcohol use, caffeine intake, and poly-drug use should be controlled for in research studies on maternal drug use. The legal drugs alcohol and tobacco appear to be more dangerous to infants than are illegal drugs. More to the point, variables such as undernourishment, distribution of calories, past health, poverty, shelter, antenatal care, and environmental factors significantly affect pregnancy outcomes and maternal health. These variables should also be accounted for in studies related to maternal health and pregnancy outcomes.

Risk Assessment

Risk labels are an integral part of the medical model of maternal health. Risk labels are intended to draw attention to populations that have poor maternal outcomes and to provide them with specialized medical attention. Maternal drug use is perceived as a risk. However, medical professionals assume that the language of risk is objective, as all scientific thought is believed to be. Risk categories are social constructions which are both artificial and unreliable, and labelling women and infants 'at risk' can have dire psychological and social consequences, especially when medical intervention removes the mother and infant from their social support systems at a time when these are needed most (Wagner, 1994). Currently, there are no medical risk-assessment systems that include the perceptions of the mothers themselves (Oakley, 1992).

Aside from the differences in subjective opinion about who is at risk and the protocol that emerges from an 'at risk' assessment, labelling women 'high risk' becomes problematic when women refuse or are unable to change their 'at risk' behaviour. Due to the social construction and labelling of women who use drugs during pregnancy as 'high risk,' women who are unable to stop using drugs or who do not want to stop using drugs during pregnancy are perceived as failing to comply with medical advice. This perception may have adverse consequences for women. The label of 'high risk' for women who use drugs during pregnancy has not led to more resources or support for mothers. Rather, it has served to reinforce unequal power relations between medical professionals and mothers. In addition, Koren argues that women are given misinformation about maternal drug use because health professionals are 'horrified by the medicolegal risks in case the woman gives birth to a malformed child' (1997, p. 14).

As well, labelling infants 'high risk' has led to the isolation and separation of infants from their mothers through lengthy confinement in hospital, social service apprehension in Canada, and criminal charges and incarceration of mothers in the United States. The label 'NAS' is recorded on public health and school records and on foster care and adoption lists. The child and parent are stigmatized, regardless of whether the label is correct. Unfortunately for mothers and infants, when medical practitioners assess risk they are usually overly cautious, and rarely remove 'high risk' labels, even if evidence to the contrary is present (Handwerker, 1994).

A recent study examined the different reporting of neonatal opiate withdrawal (NOW) in England and Wales (Morrison & Siney, 1996). Data were collected at maternity units about NOW assessment charts which list risk factors, drug treatment of withdrawal symptoms, and referral systems. One hundred and ninety-one questionnaires were returned, and it was discovered that eight different NOW assessment charts were being used by maternity units. The list of symptoms attributable to withdrawal varied on each NOW assessment chart, and different drugs were given to infants to manage withdrawal symptoms. Morrison and Siney note that many of the NOW symptoms listed on the assessment charts are subjective; in addition, many of the symptoms listed are exhibited by infants who have not been exposed to maternal drug use. Nevertheless, all symptoms exhibited by infants who are being monitored for NOW symptoms are 'often automatically attributed to withdrawal' (1996). The researchers list a number of medical problems – such as metabolic abnormalities, and mild cerebral irritation caused by foetal hypoxia and instrumentally assisted deliveries – that can mimic withdrawal symptoms in the newborn infant. It was discovered that many of the maternity units used the assessment charts for infants exposed to other (non-opiate) illicit drugs, even though there is no empirical evidence to suggest that withdrawal occurs. In summary, the risk assessment and care of infants exposed to maternal drug use is often subjective and inappropriate, and sometimes (when not clinically indicated) discriminatory.

Judges in both Canada and the United States are now asked to assess risk in maternal drug cases, and medical evidence is presented as if it is scientific fact rather than a social construction (Gómez, 1994; Handwerker, 1994). Since it is assumed that parents are unable to care for infants labelled 'high risk,' doctors are called in to testify in family court cases involving child apprehension by social services. The mother is perceived by the prosecutor as antagonistic to the foetus and to foetal outcomes. This trend encourages women to avoid medical care during pregnancy for fear of being identified as 'at risk' and made vulnerable to criminal prosecution in the United States, and child apprehension in both Canada and the United States.

Siney (1995) states that the majority of maternal drug research comes from the United States, where there is no access to health care for poor people, and that social deprivation is linked to poor maternal outcomes. These findings also illuminate the differences discovered between research findings in the United States and countries that have different socio-economic environments and drug legislation. The debate surrounding risk categories reveals the differences and assumptions underlying two models of health: the medical model and the social model. According to the medical model of health, pregnancy and birth are a medical problem where medical intervention is necessary to decrease risk of pathology and death (Wagner, 1994). The social model of health perceives birth as a biosocial process that is part of the daily fabric of life. In addition, the social model of health considers social factors that affect maternal outcomes, such as poverty, poor nutrition, lack of housing, and lack of social support.

Pregnant women want continuity of care during pregnancy that is supportive, sympathetic, and provided by other women. Indeed, it appears that this type of support is more effective than medical interventions during pregnancy (Oakley, 1992). Furthermore, woman-centred midwifery support is both safe and inexpensive (Burtch, 1994; Hepburn, 1990; Saxell, 1994; Siney, 1994, 1995; Wagner, 1994). Successful maternal services for women who use illicit drugs have striven to normalize pregnancy and birth (Siney, 1994, 1995; Hepburn, 1990, 1993a, 1993b).

It is well documented that when pregnant women are offered non-judgmental, comprehensive prenatal care and infant follow-up, maternal outcomes have improved. This is so in spite of 'high risk' categories and socio-economic status (Hepburn, 1993a, 1993b; Higgins, Moxley, Pencharz, Mikolainis, & Dubois, 1989; Latchem, 1994; Lazarus, 1988; Siney, 1994, 1995; Siney et al., 1995). Furthermore, the data consistently suggest that social environment is just as important, or more important, in infant development as prenatal exposure to drugs (Chasnoff et al., 1992; Dreher et al., 1994; Kaltenbach & Finnegan, 1989; Lifshitz, Wilson, Smith, & Desmond, 1983, 1985; Nugent, 1984). In light of the research available, neonatal abstinence syndrome appears to be a cultural fabrication.

The Method: A Feminist Perspective

Feminists have a methodological affinity with others who have written critically about drugs and who also value subjective experience. Such writers have examined the impact of race and class and the construction of language and have striven to overturn traditional views concerning licit and illicit drug use. However, until recently, they have failed to incorporate a gender analysis in their research.

Attempts to categorize and separate women who come to the attention of social services, the medical profession, and the criminal justice system from conventional society disregard the near universality of drug use and the diversity of illicit drug users. Categorization of this kind encourages one to see certain groups of people as Other. However, it is not just women who use illicit drugs who are regulated by the law, medicine, and social services. According to Smart and Smart (1978), all women experience social control. Socio-economic environment, law, and class, gender, and race mediate one's own experience of illicit drug use, and one's experience of social control.

Many feminists emphasize 'the importance of sex, race and class as factors which *together* determine the social construction of femaleness' (hooks, 1989, p. 23). Turpel (1993) notes that race, class, and gender cannot be separated, for one cannot be experienced without the others. As will be argued in this book, women's experience of illicit drug use is mediated by their race, class, and gender, in conjunction with the legal and socio-economic environment.

Feminist research embraces a dialectical method of inquiry which recognizes the relations that underlie everyday experience and the connections between the two (Acker, Barry, & Essevald, 1991, p. 135). Its aim is to create social change (Reinharz, 1992) and specifically to help transform women's lives (Jayaratne & Stewart, 1991). The researcher is part of the research (Smith, 1986; Stanley & Wise, 1979). Each interview is reflexive – a back-and-forth process that establishes rapport (Reinharz, 1992; Smith, 1986).

Hansson (1995), in discussing 'progressive-realist' criminology in South Africa, summarizes grounding principles which also apply to the type of action-research being revived among U.S. and Canadian feminists. These principles articulate my own methodological ethos:

(a) non-exploitation of those who are researched or affected by research; (b) active sharing of resources, skills and information between researchers and researched, including direct assistance to the researched where appropriate; (c) accountability of researchers to the researched; (d) active participation in the research process by those who are researched, particularly through democratic consultation about what is to be researched, how it is to be investigated and what is to be done with the knowledge that is produced; (e) the placement of researchers on the same analytical plane as the researched. (Hansson, 1995, p. 46)

In order to hear the subjective voices of women, I have chosen qualitative (inductive) research methods for this study. Open-ended interviews conducted have allowed for the movement from observation to theory and for an interpretive framework of analysis. Qualitative methods are not exclusive to feminists (see Glaser & Strauss, 1967; Jackson, 1987; Lofland & Lofland, 1984). Such methods focus on process and theory construction, a process refined by Kirby and McKenna (1989), which builds on 'grounded theory' by using constant comparisons and questioning (Glaser & Strauss, 1967; Kirby & McKenna, 1989; Strauss & Corbin, 1990). Grounded theory consists of a bottom-up, circular, up-and-down procedure where 'interpretation underlies the entire research process' (Kirby & McKenna, 1989, p. 23). Researchers attempt to formulate theory during the research process, rather than having a prior hypothesis direct the research (Glaser & Strauss, 1967; Lofland & Lofland, 1984; Strauss & Corbin, 1990). Feminists have adopted and extended qualitative research methods that emphasize triangulation or the combining of methods (Jayaratne & Stewart, 1991).

Given the lack of information concerning women's opinions about the institutions that often define and shape their lives, I have selected an interview format that facilitates the airing of opinion and the revelation of experience, rather than one that is centred on life history, ethnography,[6] or 'career.' Critical research differs from conventional research in that 'it locates specific practices in a wider social structure in an attempt to dig beneath surface appearances. It addresses myths or contradictions as expressions of oppressive social structures' (Harvey, 1990, p. 14). As a researcher, I have no need to speculate on how the legal, social service, and medical professions affect women who use illicit drugs. What is surprising is that, to date, few people have questioned illicit drug users about their opinions and suggestions regarding social policy, medical treatment, and the laws that seek to regulate and control them.

The Fieldwork and Interviews

My professional experience as a teacher, community support worker, and counsellor to women over the previous fifteen years informs this book. Unlike many researchers who choose to study a specific population, I am well acquainted with many women who had used illicit drugs but were not visible users.[7] I am also familiar with the areas of highly visible sale, distribution, and use of illicit drugs in Vancouver, B.C. Finally, I am aware of the diversity of illicit users as determined by class, race, expectations, social setting, and drug of choice. Therefore, I had no difficulty in deciding where or how to do my fieldwork. Having lived within a community where drugs were part of the daily fabric of life has given me experiential knowledge that no amount of preparation, fieldwork, or reading could have provided.

Social science research rarely acknowledges the less problematic user, or the user outside of a visible street scene. This focus on problematic and poor users as the norm has biased social research. The invisibility of other drug users has made research outside of the street scene more difficult, but not impossible. When upper- and middle-class drug users are included (see Blackwell, 1983; Cheung et al., 1991; Erickson et al., 1987; Granfield & Cloud, 1996; Matthews et al., 1995; Morgan & Joe, 1997; Sterk-Ilifson, 1996; Waldorf et al., 1991) it becomes apparent that many of the characteristics and attributes assigned to drug users by social researchers have nothing to do with the drugs, and everything do with the users' status in society (their class, race, and gender) and the illicit status of specific drugs. Hence my commitment to including interviews with women who were not visible drug users at the time of the interview.

My work with Drug and Alcohol Meeting Support for Women (DAMS)[8] in the previous five years has served to place the concerns of poor women attempting to exit a street lifestyle within the scope of this research as well. I was daily reminded of just how difficult it is for women to achieve any semblance of stability in their own lives in the absence of social and economic support. My experiences with community services and with DAMS have made me critical of the kind of policy recommended by many researchers in this area. Services and policies that are client-directed speak to the needs of the affected community, rather than the assumptions and needs of the researcher.

In addition to my fieldwork with DAMS, I spent three weeks in Europe visiting programs for women who use illicit drugs, with a special emphasis on programs for mothers. I interviewed directors, employees, and users of specific programs in Liverpool, Glasgow, Amsterdam, and Rotterdam. The interviews and fieldwork were the end result of many years of reading and correspondence regarding services available to women who used illicit drugs and their children in these areas. This research appeared to contradict policy and research results in the United States and Canada. I was curious to see these services first-hand, especially after meeting Dr Mary Hepburn, from Glasgow, when she visited DAMS in Vancouver, and Catherine Siney, a midwife from Liverpool, at a conference in Vancouver in 1993. Both of these women were providing services, and demonstrating pregnancy outcomes, that were very different from those found in North America. After corresponding with them and other professionals in the field, I decided to visit in September 1993. These contacts have created a framework for comparing different policies and treatments for women who use illicit drugs prior to and during pregnancy.

The research was approved by the Simon Fraser University Ethics Review Committee. Each participant signed a detailed consent form listing the potential risks and benefits of the study and assuring confidentiality. The interviews were semi-structured, open-ended, and of one to three hours' duration. My subjects were adult mothers in Western Canada (British Columbia, Alberta, and Saskatchewan) who have used illicit drugs. I conducted a total of twenty-eight interviews with women who were using or had used illicit drugs. All of the mothers interviewed have been given fictional names in order to preserve their anonymity.

The interview with the founding director of the Sunny Hill Hospital for Children NAS program in British Columbia is identified by a coded number. I chose to highlight the founding director at Sunny Hill, rather than other program directors outside of B.C., because the majority of the women interviewed were from British Columbia. Consequently, they were familiar with the NAS program at Sunny Hill, and I was able to juxtapose their opinions with those of the founding director.

The women interviewed were chosen through a snowball sampling. I interviewed seven women I knew and asked each one whether she knew anyone else who would like to contribute to the research. Fortunately, the snowball sampling was quite effective in including women outside of the original social network. When setting up the interview, I asked each woman if she would be willing to participate in an interview where she could give her opinions about her past or current illicit drug use. Aside from my giving some information about myself and an example of the kind of questions I would be asking, the women had no information prior to the interview.

None of the women was contacted at a clinic or in prison. Critical researchers in this field have noted that interviewing participants in prison and clinic populations may skew results (Waldorf et al., 1991). People in prisons and clinics represent only a small minority of illicit drug users – the poor, the most visible, and the most problematic. Moreover, captive participants may not be able to express themselves freely.

None of the participants was paid. The interviews took place either in the women's homes or in mine. After the first seven interviews were completed, I re-examined the interview format, made minor adjustments, noted consistencies and patterns in response, and developed a coding schedule. Over the years I had noted that women who used illicit drugs had specific concerns related to social services, the criminal justice system, and medical care for themselves and their children. Therefore, my interview schedule was constructed to reflect these interests and concerns voiced by the mothers during the interview process (see Appendix A). In order to obtain a diverse cross-section of women who use illicit drugs, I included women of different classes, ages, and races. All the women interviewed described themselves as being addicted or having a dependence on drugs, according to Alexander's (1990) continuum of involvement[9] in drug use.

I interviewed only women who had used narcotics (opiate derivatives) and/or coca derivatives (cocaine, crack) for more than one year. The mean duration of use was fourteen years. I had originally intended to interview only women who used narcotics (opiate derivatives), but I broadened my research in order to address poly-drug use and the phenomenon of 'crack babies.' Specifically, I have endeavoured to explore stereotypes and broaden the perspective of categories of drug users.

This book includes only a brief discussion of the impact of AIDS on women who use illicit drugs. During the interviews, the subject of AIDS was brought up briefly by two participants. I also was aware of several feminist research projects that address the issue of AIDS, such as that conducted by Rudd and Taylor (1992), who present oral histories of women with AIDS, as well as medical information. This study and others effectively address the concerns of women living with AIDS.

The women's responses to the interview questions were passionate and articulate. It appears that mothers who use illicit drugs have very specific views on the events that shape their lives. It may be that the women who agreed to be interviewed were more articulate than other illicit drug users. However, recent sociological studies have demonstrated that illicit drug users are informed about the social forces that shape their lives and about their own personal choices and responsibilities in relation to their illicit drug use (see Blackwell, 1983; Cheung et al., 1991; Erickson et al., 1987; Granfield & Cloud, 1996; Maher, 1995; Matthews et al., 1995; Morgan & Joe, 1997; Rosenbaum, 1981; Sterk-Ilifson, 1996; Taylor, 1993; Waldorf et al., 1991). Maher (1995) notes that there is scant evidence to demonstrate that women who use illicit drugs lie or omit information when being interviewed. Taylor (1993) and Maher (1995) also suggest that it is more difficult for participants to lie or try to make false impressions when the researcher has an ongoing relationship with them through participant observation and fieldwork. I found this to be true in my research; I have maintained an ongoing relationship with all but three of the women interviewed and it appears that they represented themselves fairly in their interviews.

The majority of the women interviewed informed me that they had never been involved in any type of social research. No one had been involved in research concerning illicit drug use. The reason they decided to participate was the fact that I was familiar with their lifestyle. They assumed that I would be sensitive to their concerns, rather than voyeuristic. Every participant was aware of my own background, and most brought my background up when introducing me to other participants within the snowball sample. My background is significant in that it may have elicited a wider range of responses than would otherwise have been obtained. As one woman (Pat) stated, 'Where you've been determines what I say to you and how I answer your questions.'[10] From this place the research project began.

A Biographical Profile

The 28 women interviewed for this study represent a wide range of life experience and biographical information. Eighty-six per cent (24) of the women lived in the Lower Mainland of B.C., and 14 per cent (4) lived in the Prairie provinces. The women ranged in age from 20 to 51; the mean age was 35. Of the 28 women interviewed, 32 per cent were women of colour – of these, 25 per cent (7) were First Nation, and 7 per cent (2) were African American. Thirty-six per cent (10) of the women were not high-school graduates; 25 per cent (7) had a high school or GED degree,

TABLE 1.1
Demographic Characteristics of Interviewees

Total Sample: 28	N	%
Age		
21–5 years	6	21
26–30 years	4	14
31–5 years	1	3
36–40 years	8	28
41–5 years	5	18
46–50 years	2	7
51+ years	2	7
Marital Status		
Single	19	68
Married/common law	7	25
Widowed	2	7
Race		
European Heritage	19	68
African American	2	7
First Nation	7	25
Education Completed		
Grades 9–11	10	36
Grades 12–13	7	25
Community college/Some university	5	18
University degree	3	11
Graduate degree (MA)		
Socio-economic Status		
Professions/managers	6	21
Self-employed/middle management	2	7
Full-time student/volunteer with		
some welfare assistance	5	18
Welfare assistance	15	53

18 per cent (5) had two to three years of university or college, 11 per cent (3) had a BA, and 11 per cent (3) had a MA. Twenty-nine per cent (8) of the women were employed full-time, 71 per cent (20) were on welfare. Of those on welfare, 18 per cent (5) were attending university or college full-time or participating in full-time volunteer work (see table 1.1).

All of the women had used either narcotics or cocaine derivatives (or both) in a dependent or addictive manner, although their drug use was not static (see table 1.2). The length of drug use varied. The mean aver-

TABLE 1.2
Children of Interviewees

Total Sample: 59	N	%
Currently in mother's custody	38	64
No longer in mother's custody	21	36
In permanent care of relatives	12	20
In permanent care of Ministry of Social Services	9	15
Children labelled NAS (all infant's mothers on social assistance)	14	24
Infants labelled NAS currently in mother's custody	6	43
In-patient NAS (Sunny Hill) infants	10	17
In permanent care of Ministry of Social Services	8	13
Total children in care at some point due to permanent and temporary child apprehension, relinquishing custody to relatives, or NAS in-patient care	32	54

age was fourteen years, but the range of use varied from two years to thirty-four years. Many of the women had ceased using drugs altogether at the time of the interview, and others had ceased use for periods of time up to five years before using again.

Only 18 per cent (5) of the biological fathers lived with the women and children in the home. Seventy-five per cent (21) of the women fully supported their children without financial assistance from the children's father. Sixty-eight per cent (19) of the women remained single parents. Twenty-five per cent (7) had steady partners (who were not the biological fathers of their children) or were married (see table 1.1). Eighteen per cent (5) stated that they were in new relationships that were not permanent.

In all, there were 59 children. Of these, 14 had been labelled NAS; 10 of the 14 had been treated at the Sunny Hill in-patient program, and 7 of these 10 infants were permanently apprehended by the Ministry of Social Services (see table 1.2). In total, 36 per cent (21) of the children were no longer in their mothers' custody, although more than half of these were in the custody of relatives or ex-husbands (see table 1.2).

2

Drugs and Mothering

Women's Perception of Illicit Drug Use

Although many women who use illicit drugs in Canada are poly-drug users, most have a drug of choice. Individuals who consume drugs have varied reasons for doing so, and people can have different experiences with similar drugs (Alexander, 1990; O'Hare, 1992; Peele & Brodsky, 1991; Weil & Rosen, 1993). For example, some people prefer heroin; others prefer cocaine. For women who use illicit drugs such as heroin and cocaine, the secrecy, social stigma, and lifestyle involved can be problematic. Social attitudes regarding illicit drug use, especially in relation to mothering, are quite negative and have significant consequences for women (Humphries et al., 1992; Maher, 1992, 1995; Rosenbaum, 1981; Rosenbaum, Murphy, Irwin, & Watson, 1990; Taylor, 1993).

Researchers have noted that women's experience of illicit drugs use is often positive (Henderson, 1993a, 1993b; Rosenbaum, 1981; Taylor, 1993). The majority of the women interviewed stated that their experience of their drug use had been positive, especially when they initially began to experiment with illicit drug use. Furthermore, even the women who experienced problematic and negative addiction agreed that there were positive elements to their illicit drug use. In fact, when I asked if there had been anything positive about their drug use, they often laughed, exclaiming, 'Of course!' [Hope] and 'Oh, absolutely!' [Donna].

There seemed to be agreement among the women interviewed that illicit drug use was educational and fun. The following quotation captures the general response of the women interviewed to the question 'Has there been anything positive about your drug use?'

Initially it was exciting and fun, even educational. [Carol]

Another women noted that her drug use was fun and taught her to be a survivor:

It was fun. I really had a lot of fun in the beginning. And it taught me [that] I'm a real survivor, and a real go-getter. I'm amazed myself with the amount of money and drugs that I could come up with. [Bobbi]

A third woman explained how she would not have met all of her close friends if she had not started using illicit drugs:

Of course it was fun! I wouldn't have met all of you guys if I hadn't used. [Sarah]

One mother described the lifestyle, and her wish to live outside of the mainstream:

I loved the separate aspect of the lifestyle – sleep all day, party all night, not working but having lots of money. For example, we paid cash for a new car, took trips, etc. I had come from a poor family so I feel this played a part. I wanted to be different, out of the mainstream. I see all aspects of my life as positive as they are simply part of the process of my journey. [Carol]

Drug use, especially addiction, can be painful (Rosenbaum, 1981); however, the women interviewed described how even though they had experienced pain as a result of their addiction to illicit drugs, there were positive outcomes subsequent to their drug use. One woman describes how she learned more about herself by examining her negative addiction:

But as far as positive ... I guess I learned about compassion for people who are on drugs or alcohol. Or even have emotional hang-ups. Because I learned that my addiction [is] a symptom of my pain. Maybe I would never have learned that without the problems that I had. [Bobbi]

Another woman noted that her addiction to illicit drugs had enabled her to stay sane in the face of abuse:

I really froze after my mother died. And that was probably when my problems started, and it wasn't the drugs. The drugs were a vent. And when I was abused it

TABLE 2.1
Drug of Choice

Mean duration of use: 14 years	N	%
Total Sample: 28		
Opiate derivatives	12	43
Cocaine derivatives	11	39
Both cocaine and opiates	4	14
Talwin & Ritalin	1	3

was more of a vent. And I probably would have gone crazy if I hadn't been running away to freedom ... The drugs really kept my brain intact, and it probably kept me going through a lot of stuff; it just sort of blotted out reality for enough time so I could pick myself up again. And it really had to be [to] the point where I didn't need to blot reality out [before] I could stop. If I had stopped before then I would have just started the next time I needed it. [Donna]

For the women interviewed, drugs and drug use meant different things. Traditional drug research has ignored the positive aspects of drug use (Hadaway, Beyerstein, & Youdale, 1991; Henderson, 1993a, 1993b). Depicting female drug users solely as victims who lack agency is faulty (Henderson, 1993a, 1993b; Maher, 1995; Taylor, 1993). Similarly, describing female drug users solely as using drugs to cope with the stresses of their life is faulty (Maher, 1995). The women interviewed in this study, and in Taylor's (1993) and Maher's (1995) studies, did not conform to the prevailing stereotype of women illicit drug users as passive victims. There is a wide range of responses to illicit drug use.

The Drug of Choice?

Of the women interviewed for this study, 3 per cent used Ts & Rs (Talwin and Ritalin), 43 per cent considered themselves to be narcotic users (users of opiate derivatives), 39 per cent were cocaine users, and 14 per cent used narcotics and cocaine equally (see table 2.1). At the time of the interview, 25 per cent of the women were taking legal methadone (see table 5.2). Thirty-six per cent had been on legal methadone in the past.

All of the women interviewed had strong opinions about their drugs of choice and their preference for regular use. All had experimented with both stimulants and depressants and with poly-drug use. In contrast with the disease models of addiction, it was clear that their experiences differed in terms of both physiological effects of the drugs and patterns of use. For example, the women described the different effects they experienced when using heroin and cocaine:

Coke, yes. I think that is the devil's drug. It makes you run out ... in the street and do stupid shit for it, unlike heroin. I mean, I used heroin for many years and I never did as many stupid things to get it as I did for coke. But I think that partially that is the nature of the drug, too. You know, you are down and out and you are pretty unaware of things going on around you and so you don't participate in them. So, in itself it keeps you safe. With heroin, at least it [lasts] six or seven hours, if it is real good. When [using cocaine] you are driven out on the street every twenty minutes. [Pat]

I think they tend to lump every drug together, too. You know, the effects of cocaine and heroin are very different. Almost total opposites, I would think. [Diane]

The route of administration, type of drug, duration of effect, and cost mediate a person's drug use. So do class, race, gender, and drug legislation. The effects of heroin generally last from four to six hours, the effects of cocaine from twenty to forty-five minutes. Therefore the type of drug used, as well as drug legislation, may mediate how the drug is experienced by the user. Not all of the women perceived cocaine as the 'devil's drug.' Rather, many who were cocaine users described their drug use in terms of their own subjective experiences and often in terms of their rejection of opiate derivatives:

Well, I never really liked junk anyway. I always got sick. I liked the go-fast drugs. But, I love the cocaine. [Sarah]

I don't like heroin. I'm not a downer. I like the rush of cocaine. I'm a speed freak. [Janet]

I had been addicted to heroin when I was sixteen ... I got off it ... I thought, oh god, I never want to go through that again. And then I was introduced to cocaine ... I think I liked that awake high much better than that sleepy [one] ... It was fun, you talked a lot. It was energy. I liked the energy. [Bobbi]

I even tried heroin ... But I didn't like the high, I didn't like sleeping ... I didn't want to be down, I wanted to be up. So cocaine was the thing. [Ellie]

The women who preferred cocaine to heroin use were attracted to its stimulating effects. In addition, one young woman noted that she felt her drug use was more in control with cocaine than with heroin:

When you are on heroin you get sick. You have to do it. And I didn't like that idea of, you know, the drug was controlling me, and I didn't want to be under that much control. [Karen]

Obviously, heroin and cocaine are not as compelling as once thought. The women in this study tried many different drugs without becoming addicted to them. It is evident that many individuals experiment with heroin and cocaine use without becoming long-term users (Blackwell, 1983; Cheung, Erickson, & Landau, 1991; Erickson, Adlaf, Murray, & Smart, 1987; Matthews, Dawes, Nadeau, Wong, & Alexander, 1995; Waldorf, Reinarman, & Murphy, 1991).

In contrast to the women who preferred cocaine or other stimulants, many of the women who preferred heroin described cocaine use in negative terms. Two women from working-class backgrounds stated:

I never did like cocaine all that much, though I did it because it was there ... But it was not my drug of choice ever and I was always really afraid of the come down. [I] hated the whole scene, it was such a mess. People would o.d. [overdose], and all those needles, and all the blood, yuk; and all those misses ... oh god. [Gloria]

I did every drug ... the only drug I never did was crack ... I could have done crack too, but somewhere I heard that they use ... some kind of cleaning thing to do it, and I thought I'm not doing that ... I wouldn't do it, I thought of it as bad for my health [laughter]. [Morgan]

The fact that cocaine needs to be injected or sniffed more often than heroin, due to the short duration of its effect, changes the environment of use for many women, especially intravenous (IV) users. For the majority of women, their drug of choice depended on assessment of risk and whether they preferred a stimulant effect or a depressant effect. However, many who preferred depressants noticed that, once they became addicted to heroin, it began to have an energizing effect. For example, one professional woman described how she cleaned house after using heroin:

Instead of doing what they're meant to do, they do the opposite. So I know there's metabolic changes going on or whatever [laughter] ... it was wonderful to be high to do housework. I would have all this energy. Well, you are supposed to be on the nod. I mean when you are first using, sure you nod out. I couldn't move or I would throw up. I don't know why I continued doing it. But the thing is, when you do it often you do it for energy. [Gloria]

While using heroin, women found that household chores became more bearable, and regular use altered the effects of heroin. Many of the women noted that heroin was their preferred drug:

I got into heroin so quick, actually ... before anything else. I just left everything else. Then it was just heroin. [Evelyn]

Heroin or opium is my drug of choice, but smoking it now. [Hope]

I was more like a chippy; I mean I chipped every day. [Sarah]

I loved opiates right from the beginning, and recognized that I could get opiates in other forms, other than opium and smoking it. So I was able to start figuring out how to do codeine, how to do pills every day, that kind of stuff. [Debbie]

All of the women were self-educated about the numerous legal drugs they could consume. The wide array of pharmaceutical drugs available contributed to their poly-drug use, especially when heroin was scarce and expensive. Some of the women whose drug of choice was heroin used methadone, legal narcotics, and heroin interchangeably, according to availability. Licit drugs were very much a part of the women's overall drug consumption.

Many of the women discussed their own use, and the use of their family of origin, of legal drugs. Tobacco, alcohol, and pharmaceutical drugs formed a backdrop to their discussion of illicit drug use. However, the fact that many illicit drug users are poly-drug users does not mean that all drugs are interchangeable, or wanted. One woman who has been on legal methadone for over fifteen years noted:

I never did a Valium. In fact I rarely even did aspirin. [Evelyn]

Other women noted:

I know that my drug of choice is not coffee, because I'm different from most people because I don't like coffee. And I get high from coffee, and it's not pleasant. [Morgan]

I don't like methadone personally. I felt like this is the only drug that they would allow to be legal. [Hope]

If I had a choice of how I wanted to get high it wouldn't be a beer. [Morgan]

This is my one habit [cigarettes] that I allow myself to keep without guilt ... I mean I shouldn't have to, but I do. I know it is a big thing ... It is really way worse than any drug that I quit. [Mary]

One upper-middle-class woman explained:

When I was growing up, girls from our side of the tracks did not drink. We never drank. [Janet]

All of the women had formed opinions about specific drugs, and in practice avoided many drugs. Although some of the women had difficulty in relation to alcohol use, many of the older women rejected alcohol, perceiving it as the drug of choice of their parents:

So all of that generation smoked cigarettes and drank heavily and the following generation, which was my generation, we were all heavy [drug] users. [Debbie]

Still, many of the women recognized that even though they had chosen illicit drugs, they were following the same path as their parents in terms of their dependent use of a drug. One woman from a middle-class background stated:

Alcohol has never been a problem ... But I was raised by a severely alcoholic family, and we never wanted to have anything to do [with alcohol]. I kept fighting. I am not going to be like my mother. I am not going to be like my mother. But I am. [Pat]

However, the legal availability of alcohol makes it significantly different from heroin and cocaine. Whereas it is socially unacceptable for women to drink heavily in North America (Addiction Research Foundation, 1996, p. 31; Sandmaier, 1980), the criminalization of women who use illicit drugs involves much heavier penalties.

Social Attitudes and Social Stigma

During the interviews many of the women described prevalent social attitudes concerning illicit drug use. Misconceptions and stereotypes were
discussed, as well as the consequences of misinformation regarding illicit
drug use. One prevalent myth equates all illicit drug use with highly visible street use. Many of the women described how this misconception
affected them:

One worker says, well, did you ever go downtown? Everyone associated downtown
... I guess you can call us ... suburban junkies. [Evelyn]

People think that addicts are easily identifiable or maybe they don't, I don't know.
But there seems to be a consensus [that] they are only on the street; that's just not
true. When I went to the treatment centre there were sixty-year-old women kick-
ing Valium addiction, narcotics addictions for painkillers that they had for arthritis, or whatever, you know. Whatever it started out to be, they got wired out on the
painkiller. And they are getting them, not for killing the pain of arthritis but
because they were sick without them. [Gloria]

Where a person consumes her drug and how she obtains it depends on
her socio-economic status[1] and on drug legislation. Middle- and upper-
class users do not have to buy on the street; rather, they are able to obtain
illicit drugs in their own neighbourhoods:

It wasn't hard to find. It was like every neighbourhood had the neighbourhood
house dealer ... I was never downtown ... Never had to. [Evelyn]

In addition, the social fiction separating illicit drug users from users of
prescribed legal pharmaceuticals was apparent to the women interviewed. Alexander (1990) notes how negative labels reserved for illicit
drug users have emerged in North America. All of the women, regardless
of socio-economic status, were aware of the negative stereotyping of illicit
drug users in Canada. Stereotypes made it difficult for many of the
women to reveal their illicit drug use to others, and sometimes even to
come to terms with their own illicit drug use. The women stated that most
illicit drug users were perceived as 'addicts' rather than as individual
women who use illicit drugs, and their humanity was obscured:

It's like the war on drugs has made a monster out of this. And they are not willing to look at people as individuals and as human beings with problems and with circumstances in their lives that are even external to the drug use. [Carol]

Yeah, you are not a person, you are just an alcoholic or you are a drug user. [Cindy]

You know, in many ways drug addicts are extremely good scapegoats for North Americans. I mean we don't have scapegoats, we can't use religion now. We can't use colour now. What is there left? ... So we use drug users and street people. [Theresa]

Maybe some people have this thing inside where they have to feel better than you. I don't know, I've heard people say that. And especially in the white, dominant society ... Is it true that these people want to oppress another group? Or have a need to do that? ... I don't think that that's a natural feeling, but I think that's what's happening. And I classify drug addicts right in there with other oppressed groups: women, people of colour, even handicapped people. [Morgan]

Alexander (1990) states that the 'the war on drugs' fits the same pattern of wars of persecution. The connection between social attitudes and personal use of illicit drugs was relevant to the women interviewed. They were conscious of the larger social, political, and economic variables that not only shaped their personal drug use, but contributed to their oppression and to that of other groups outside the dominant white culture. The women questioned the prevailing environment that perpetuated oppression. One professional woman stated:

You know, sometimes I wake up, hear something on the news and I wonder what kind of society is this? What have we created? It's so horrific, it's so twisted. The other night some hockey team won and cars were beeping and people shouting for over an hour. All that passion for a hockey game. But try to interest people in changing society – looking at war, for instance. Even the peace march was cancelled this year for lack of participation. Now what kind or society is that? I really don't understand how people ... can be so ignorant, so blind. Why don't they get it that this whole segment of society is being trashed? They think they're outside of it. But this attitude of wanting to judge, control, and hurt drug users is sick. You can't turn on the TV, or watch a movie, without seeing some drug dealer blown away. Even in books there's all these references to 'drug addicts.' What's so frightening to me is these references assume that it is something criminal, deviant, evil, less than. These aren't people any more, they don't even have names, just 'dealer' or 'addict' and we are all supposed to know what that means. Well, I don't. There is a person under all that. [Hope]

The social, political, and economic environment shapes illicit drug use. Furthermore, the limiting and oppressive structure of society can often become glaringly apparent when one's behaviour is criminalized.

Just as traditional drug literature presents a prevalence of negative (as opposed to positive) motivations for illicit drug use, negative stereotypes regarding illicit drug users prevail among the public. Yet, most of the women interviewed described other users in positive terms. Often it was a person or group of people, rather than the drugs themselves, that brought women to associate with other individuals who used illicit drugs. For example, several women noted:

Yeah, the people I liked were doing drugs, although they were doing soft drugs. [Gloria]

Even when I first starting using drugs, for the first time, illegal drugs, the people who I did them with were great; they were nice people. [Morgan]

I think addicts are the most loving, caring people that you could ever meet. [Sarah]

We got support amongst the other addicts. I mean we became good friends ... not because we are just addicts together, but we had something more in common. You know, ... we like what we are doing but, you know, the lifestyle that goes with it, is what we didn't like ... But, other than that, I ended up with the best friends ... Yes. I still see them. You know, to this day they are still supportive ... You know, even though our lives have gone different directions, all of us. But ... our friends were our support. That is when true friendship really came about ... they say a junkie doesn't have friends. That is not true. [Evelyn]

And of course it turned out that these were just normal people and I liked them and I thought, well, I feel fine here. This can't be so terrible. And I don't regret that. [Linda]

For many of the women, the stereotype of the deviant addict was quickly abandoned once they met illicit drug users. Similar to other studies of female drug users (Rosenbaum, 1981; Taylor, 1993), in place of stereotypical negative characteristics, they found lasting friendship and support. They recognized the thin line separating users and non-users:

You [society] think that you are so much different than I am, that I am a breed apart, but I am the same person you are. And I have been on your side and I have been on my side. And I know how easy it is to jump from one to the other, and how easy it could happen to you. [Pat]

However, women crossed the line separating licit and illicit drug use, the illegal status of their drug of choice had significant ramifications, especially in terms of lifestyle.

Lifestyle

The life of an illicit drug user can be very difficult, especially if she is poor. Besides her fear of arrest and child apprehension, there is the constant need for money to buy drugs on the illegal market. Many of the women, both low-income and middle-class, discussed the lifestyle that often accompanies the use of criminalized drugs:

I really hope people don't choose this path. I wouldn't wish it on anybody, you know ... It's just too hard. It's always a problem. [Gloria]

It has affected my life very detrimentally by having to see certain people that I would not necessarily see, because of course that has been part of my life ... who has got, and who has got stolen stuff ... you know, the whole criminal stuff. [I'm] subjected to [that] constantly. [Judy]

Yeah, it is mostly the bizarre nature of the lifestyle ... I couldn't live with it any more. It was making me crazy. [Pat]

The criminalization of drugs contributes to the illegal market that women must negotiate in order to buy illicit drugs. In this environment they often have limited choices in whom they buy their drugs from. As well, although they may be able to maintain a fairly stable environment within their homes, negotiating to buy and sell drugs has often brought the women in contact with other criminal activity and police surveillance (Taylor, 1993). However, the majority of women were adamant that it was not their illicit drug use that was wrong, but social attitudes and poverty that contributed to an unpredictable lifestyle:

Give me a break. I mean, you take something as innocuous as drugs and turn around and say 'Oh, this is terrible,' when it is society that makes the life terrible. Not the drugs themselves. [Theresa]

Other women noted that financial status strongly affected their experiences as illicit drug users. One professional woman from a working-class background stated:

Even when you are using, that's not all you're doing. You still have a life, relationships, goals. The poorer you are the more time it takes to get money to score. But if you have money, or the drugs, it doesn't take that much time to use. So you are just living your life the rest of the time. [Hope]

Another professional woman noted:

At that time, because of the success of my drug dealing ... I was able to easily get money, easily keep myself in supply. [Debbie]

And one mother who had been a full-time university student noted:

I didn't lead a life where I had to do terrible things ... I was never really hungry and I never had to be a prostitute unless I felt like it. You know, I was sick a few times but generally I had drugs and had money and, as a matter of fact, I was way better off financially than I have been since I've gone to school. [Theresa]

Illicit drug use is just one variable in a woman's life. The time and energy devoted to obtaining drugs is determined in part by one's class. Street use usually involves daily buying and selling of drugs, often several times a day, as one earns the money through legal and illegal activities. Other less visible use is shaped by the larger quantities of drugs available. Many middle- and upper-class users in this study were able to buy and sell large quantities of drugs. Such women did not have to devote time and energy to the daily acquisition of their drugs of choice the way a street user would have to. Therefore, similiar to Morgan and Joe's (1997) findings, the pattern of use and selling drugs shifts according to availability and economic status.

Prominent themes running through the interviews included the lack of legitimacy, silencing, and social stigma attached to illicit drug use. The term 'social stigma' refers to negative labels 'affixed to the social image of individuals or groups, and which, ... serve as a means of social control' (Shoham & Hoffman, 1991, p. 106). The social stigma attached to illicit drug use was described by low-income, middle-class, and professional women:

Just the misinformation that goes out about drugs and drug use to the public ... people form their immediate opinion of anyone that's used drugs ... I think that's been the worst thing for me, that stigma. That I've managed to repress myself as an adult because of things I did years ago ... low self-esteem, all of that. Basically what it did for me, the laws have attached a stigma to drug use ... And that's really hard to get over ... if you ever do get over it. [Morgan]

Heroin ... [there's] so much of a social stigma on it. [Linda]

Another myth that really irritates me is the one [that] every junkie is out selling to the kids in the street and the schools. I mean, it is just not true. Yes, there are some really sleazy people. Probably in ... larger urban centres where there is a lot more access to drugs. Like maybe in Vancouver. [But] I don't think that is happening. When I lived in Vancouver, I never saw it ... the police love to have everybody think that is true, because that makes everybody hate us. I mean, we are the dregs of the earth. Definitely ... who is worse than a junkie, nobody. And who is worse than a junkie mother? I mean that is the ultimate put down, right? ... all it is to me, is just the ultimate in sadness. [Carol]

The worst thing you can be in this society is a drug addict or a drug pusher. I think it is a harder thing to overcome than being a murderer. When you look at sentences, people who traffic drugs ... I am talking about people who traffic, who are addicts and who are trafficking to keep themselves going. They end up with more time than people who molest children ... And they did more time, a greater percentage of their sentence than people who do other things. Now, I think that ... this society has done a really good job of misleading the public ... laying out all kinds of misinformation ... I think that our society has to get real about it ... even if they do decriminalize it, well they won't decriminalize it unless some of these things and attitudes get changed ... Basically, they are making it impossible for a lot of people to ever get beyond this. I think that they think that people [who] become addicted are weak and stupid ... I think that a lot of people end up believing that they are. Even if you are really strong ... sometimes, it is just really hard to get out and to get beyond this. [Diane]

We ourselves are not bad people and we have to look at that first. Because when they treat you like shit, then you react like shit. You know, if you treat me a certain way, then I am going to react to that. But, I also don't think that drug users need sympathy all the time. We just need to be treated like human beings. [Sarah]

The social stigma surrounding illicit drug use takes a personal toll on women (Ettorre, 1992; Rosenbaum, 1981; Rosenbaum et al., 1990; Taylor, 1993), for the negative images are difficult to challenge in one's private and public life, whether one is a visible or a non-visible illicit drug user. The barrage of negative images reinforces both stereotypes and harsh drug policy and legislation. All of this contributes to an environment of dehumanizing behaviour towards illicit drug users.

Silencing and Lack of Legitimacy

All personal use of illicit drugs eventually intersects with social attitudes surrounding drug use. Even non-visible users interviewed were affected by the negative images of illicit drug users portrayed by the media and government. Often negative messages were internalized by the women, which hindered their own stabilization and recovery. Two women from working-class backgrounds conclude:

I think it's how we view people, and that's the way that I carry it. I think it's what we believe ... if ... people on the street think that they are doing a terrible thing, then they are ... Oh yeah, internalize it and we become repressive to ourselves. And most of the damage I've done is to myself, but with the help of the entire society. But I'm the one who is there with myself and who is repressive. [Morgan]

Even people that are your friends and love you, it's hard for them to understand because we're bombarded by the media and by ... the whole attitude, the whole ... Christian sort of [attitude] like good/bad ... or weak/strong. But even within ourselves we feel that, right. So you can't really blame other people for falling into that pattern of thinking about you. [Gloria]

Trying to maintain a positive identity in relation to illicit drug use can be very difficult in the face of opposition. Furthermore, the secrecy involved in illicit drug use furthers one's sense of alienation from mainstream culture and from one's immediate friends and family. Three professional women note:

Being a drug addict is almost like being a baby-rapist or something. The way people see you ... I just hate the secrecy ... I hate to have to hide, I really do. But I have to ... I think, if only I hadn't taken that path. It closed some paths forever, or it seems to. I don't know if that is true but I feel like there are some doors forever closed to me. [Gloria]

I have always felt that; that is a part of my life that I have been forced to hide. And even throughout my recovery like ... I am not comfortable to share that with people, because I know that it will be taken in a negative way. I am afraid of the ramifications. I worked so hard to get where I am that ... I think that it would be beneficial, I would love to share my past and have it in a positive light, so that it is a role model for other people ... When I was addicted, there was nobody out there that I could say, well, they made it. Because the way that it is all set up is that you only look at the negative things. You only look at the people who are going back to jail. I mean, just turn on the news any night. [Carol]

The stigma and the secrecy [are] really difficult. At this point in my life I worry that my past will jeopardize my plans for the future ... I feel dishonest hiding my past. It feeds into that whole feeling that you are not legitimate and I had enough of that feeling when I was using. [Hope]

Not only did the need for secrecy contribute to a sense of personal dishonesty, it also reinforced the women's sense of lack of legitimacy. Secrecy and silence were essential practices to most drug users as their drugs of choice are illegal. The fear of arrest, social service intervention, social ostracism, and limited employment choices fuelled the need to remain silent. Because of the criminalization of drugs, low-income and middle-class and professional women noted that they had no legitimate voice in society:

They never ask anybody's opinion; they just go ahead and do things based on what they think but they never ask us. Nobody ever asked me what I thought. [Karen]

Indirectly, it makes you feel like some ... not a real citizen of the country ... You don't feel legitimate, a legitimate person, because you are considered a criminal. [Judy]

It is frustrating. You know, I have all this knowledge and nobody wants to listen ... The people who should listen don't want your input. Your input makes sense. Theirs doesn't. [Evelyn]

You get treated like an idiot ... that doesn't have a voice. [Pat]

I think I've been silenced all my life, through fear, by men, by society. All my life these thoughts circled around inside. No one ever took the time to ask what I thought. All these things that affect you, but no one asked. But I'm still silenced, because I'm not going to inform any public meeting or place that I'm a drug user. Let's be realistic; it's illegal to use certain drugs in our society. [Hope]

Few illicit drug users have a legitimate voice in Canada. Unlike other countries, such as the Netherlands where the Junkiebond, an interest group established in 1977 and comprising drug users, ex-users, and non-users, advocates for illicit drug users, Canada has no central organizing group of illicit drug users and ex-users representing and advocating for themselves. However, groups such as the Concerned Citizens Drug Study and Education Society in Burnaby, British Columbia, have focused on education, and more recently this focus has been expanded to challenge changes in methadone drug treatment in B.C.

Women have historically had limited participation or voice in political and private life. Criminalized women are even more circumscribed and are rarely offered a legitimate voice in society. The social stigma surrounding, and criminalization of, illicit drug use have contributed to the silencing of women. Until recently there was little information regarding female illicit drug users. Currently, much of the research on illicit drugs centres on women's failure to mother adequately, and the harm they may inflict on their unborn foetuses (Cain, 1994; Logli, 1990; Shaw, 1985; Steinberg, 1994; Williams & Bruce, 1994). The combination of mothering and illicit drug use is portrayed as immoral and dangerous. Consequently, women – and especially mothers – are seen as more deviant than their male counterparts, and this stereotype contributes to their silencing.

Illicit Drug Use and Mothering

The ideology of mothering in Western countries portrays women as virtuous, caring, giving, and pure (Collins, 1994; Glenn, 1994; Gupta, 1995). This ideology obscures the reality of mothers' daily lives. Glenn (1994) explores how women in Western society have full responsibility for family life: they are expected to take care of the household, raise the children, and care for relatives, including husbands. For most women, especially poor women, this means long hours of unpaid and unacknowledged work (Glenn, 1994; Oakley, 1986, 1992). When women are perceived by the legal, medical, or social service professions as failing in their role as mothers, they are punished (Chunn, 1995; Gallagher, 1987; Humphries et al., 1992; Maher, 1992; Maier, 1992; Rosenbaum et al., 1990). When women are denied the chance to mother their own children through separation as a result of incarceration or child apprehension, they are further stigmatized by society through social ostracism and harsh sentencing (Carlen, 1976, 1983; Daly, 1987; Eaton, 1983, 1985; Masson, 1992).

Women who use illicit drugs are considered to be unfit mothers, out of control, and a danger to their children (Paltrow, 1992; Rosenbaum et al., 1990; Taylor, 1993). However, a comparable set of characteristics concerning fathers who use illicit drugs is lacking in drug literature. Although most research on illicit drug use centres on the male user, his parenting qualities and responsibility to his family are rarely addressed. Rather, the male user has often been described as the 'man about town' (Preble & Casey, 1969), and little was known about his family relations until Hanson, Beschner, Walters, and Bovelle (1985) studied male heroin users in the United States. Outside of the area of monetary support, little attention has been given to the family responsibilities of male illicit drug users. This reflects Western ideological assumptions about men, as opposed to ideological assumptions concerning women.

In contrast, research on women who use illicit drugs overwhelmingly explores, and often centres on, the women's lack of parenting abilities, and failure to be responsible for children and the household (see Chasnoff, 1989; Dembo et al., 1990; Densen-Gerber & Rohrs, 1973; Howard, Beckwith, Rodning, & Kropenske, 1989; Jaudes, Ekwo, & Voorhis, 1995; Julien, 1992; Kantor, 1978; Murphy et al., 1991; Peak & Papa, 1993; Robins & Mills, 1993; Steinberg, 1994; Weston, Ivins, Zuckerman, Jones, & Lopez, 1989).

However, as noted earlier, on reviewing the literature on mothers who use illicit drugs, it becomes apparent that qualitative research with in-depth interviews (see Colten, 1980, 1982; Dreher, Nugent, & Hudgins, 1994; Jackson & Berry, 1994; Kearney, Murphy, & Rosenbaum, 1994; Leeders, 1992; Rosenbaum, 1981; Rosenbaum et al., 1990; Sterk-Elifson, 1996; Taylor, 1993) demonstrate that these mothers can be adequate parents and view mothering as their central role.

For many women, pregnancy is an event that significantly changes their status in society (Kitzinger, 1992; Oakley, 1992; Rothman, 1989). Women who are identified as illicit drug users during pregnancy are closely monitored by medical and social services professionals, who assess, and eventually determine, maternal health and parental fitness.

In the course of the research, it became apparent that the women interviewed perceived themselves as different from male drug users who are parents, because of their role as mothers. The full responsibility of caring for their children shaped their drug use, both positively and negatively. Women in Canadian society are offered little socio-economic support in caring for their families, and when family break-up occurs the individual mother is blamed rather than society. Caring for children and other family members is difficult, time-consuming work. Many of the women spoke about the sole responsibility of mothering when responding to question 8, 'Has it been different for you being a mother who uses drugs than, say, a male drug user?' Eighty-nine per cent of the women claimed that their role as mothers who used illicit drugs was different from that of male users. The sole responsibility for care and the lack of fathers' participation in the family were evident in their responses:

The whole idea of having a child, to be a mother, to take care of and support that child and love him. I mean all those things that come with the mother category, right. You can't be out there partying and hanging out, and coming home when you want to. Being stable and having a home and cooking meals three times a day, and if you are going to school or work, well, having a good babysitter. [Ellie]

I do think men don't have the same kind of ... that's sexist too, but most men are not as committed parents. [Judy]

Oh, the twins' father was out of control, but he was a user too. He didn't have any obligations. When I would take off ... he would be in my place where I had all my kids. And the first thing he would do is phone his mother. She would come to get the kids, and then half the time he would end up downtown with me because he would know that I would have money, be making money there. He had no obligations, he basically had free rent when he wanted to come and didn't have to do anything. Being a single male he had nothing stopping him. [Donna]

Most definitely ... I guess I felt some kind of responsibility. I am not sure men always feel that responsibility as we do. [Sarah]

I have more responsibilities. A guy can split and do whatever he wants ... A woman can't. I mean, she can, but there is a bond between your children that just ... for me is unbreakable. I could not just get up and leave my kids. I may threaten them with 'You know, if you want to ... go to a foster home, you are headed in the right direction kid.' ... You know how kids get at twelve ... But I mean there is just no way ... you are bound with an unbreakable thread ... I don't know how it works. [Theresa]

Probably only for the women involved [laughter]. [Pat]

The only thing that would be different for me doing drugs, was my kids ... a man can walk away. A mother has ... no other choice, if she has a kid ... A woman can ... up and leave. But, ... who ... is going to look after the children? ... Then the mother has that guilty conscience of leaving the children behind. [Men] they don't have a conscience. [Julie]

Women felt responsible for the care of their children. Taylor (1993) notes that few of the women in her study of illicit drug users in Glasgow received help from their male partners in caring for the family, and over half of the mothers in Kearney, Murphy, and Rosenbaum's (1994) research were single parents. Similarly, in this study, the biological fathers of the children gave little or no support to the majority of the women in caring for the family. Creating and maintaining a home life, daily structure, food, shelter, and emotional and financial support were the sole responsibility of the majority of mothers. The mothers adhered to prevailing ideological assumptions about mothering and strove to maintain homes for their children. Only five of the women interviewed had supportive husbands, though three of these husbands had served lengthy prison sentences due to their status as illicit drug users, which left the mothers coping with the household without their daily support during their incarceration. In fact, the majority of the women's assessment of men in relation to family responsibility was fairly negative. As one woman of European heritage concludes,

I don't think that is common to drug-abusing people though. I mean ... all men do that, find it very easy to abandon their children. To whatever situation that they probably have little or no knowledge about and are fine to just waltz off with that ... I think that is the thing that is common to men, whether they are using drugs or drinking or doing anything else. Men are just like that ... and women aren't in general. [Pat]

For this sample of women, the majority of men offered no support and appeared to have little difficulty abandoning their families, leaving the mothers with sole responsibility for the children and household.

Pregnancy and Birth

Taking responsibility for both household and children was primary to the women interviewed. Additionally, pregnancy and birth were significant in their lives. Pregnancy, birth, and mothering are often perceived by the medical, social service, and legal professions as incompatible with illicit drug use (Cain, 1994; Logli, 1990; Shaw, 1985; Steinberg, 1994; Stone, Salerno, Green, & Zelson, 1971; Streissguth, Grant, Ernst, & Phipps, 1994; Williams & Bruce, 1994). The medical profession perceives the pregnant women and her developing foetus as being in an antagonistic relationship (Chavkin, 1992; Handwerker, 1994) and the mother is viewed as incapable of making decisions concerning her pregnancy and unreliable in reporting symptoms (Oakley, 1986). In contrast, the data presented in this section suggest that mothers are initially willing and capable of making decisions about their pregnancies.

Pregnancy and birth are biological and social acts experienced by many women. The act of becoming a mother is a social transformation that has far-reaching consequences due to societal expectations concerning mothering (Kitzinger, 1992). Women are held personally responsible by the obstetric community for the outcomes of their pregnancies (Nsiah-Jefferson, 1989). The majority of medical professionals perceive illicit drug use during pregnancy as a medical problem rather than a social problem. Therefore, women are rarely offered social supports that could contribute to a healthier pregnancy. The fact that women who use illicit drugs during pregnancy are labelled 'at risk' can have 'detrimental psychological and social consequences' for the women (Wagner, 1994, p. 34). Such labelling is artificial and unreliable, and removes women from their social support systems at a time when these are most needed (Wagner, 1994). Many of the mothers interviewed were treated poorly by the medical community during their pregnancy, and their birth experiences were less than positive.

The decision to carry a pregnancy to term is difficult for many women. Faced with the financial and emotional burden of a dependent child, the stigma associated with illicit drug use, and possible intervention by social service and medical professionals, each of the mothers interviewed perceived her pregnancies according to her own subjective assessment of the risks involved. For some, abortion was a choice. For others pregnancy offered a new start. One young Native mother on social assistance stated:

So I went out and got a test, so then I knew I was pregnant. And then right away I quit smoking because I wanted to have a baby. I wanted to have a baby that was clean. I wanted to start a new life. I didn't want to carry [on] in the tracks of my mother, you know. And I had all this burden on my shoulders ... I didn't screw

up. I didn't drink. I didn't smoke. I didn't drink coffee. I didn't eat chocolate. I didn't do anything. So it was a great big turnaround, you know ... First of
all ... I just did it for my baby ... now I'm doing it for myself. [Sue]

For the majority of the mothers, pregnancy presented conflicting choices
and limitations. Two young women note:

I didn't care about my life ... or what happened. Then I found out I was pregnant and I was going to have a ... child. I thought, well, this is something to live
for. Then I felt bad, that I was doing drugs two months into my pregnancy. So
then I prayed to god, 'Please, god, make her a normal child.' And she was fine.
[Cindy]

She won't be saying, 'Oh you used to be a drug addict, you used to do this' ...
I'll just be mummy. I get to start all over. [Karen]

Although some of the women saw their pregnancy as an opportunity to
stop using drugs, many were more realistic about the obstacles they were
facing. Some were challenged by medical professionals when they discovered they were pregnant:

I was four and a half months pregnant, and the doctor ... says, 'Well, Mrs D., you
are pregnant.' And before I could go 'yippee!' he says, 'Would you like me to
arrange for an abortion?' Just bang, nine years of waiting and that's what he
says, would you like me to arrange for an abortion. [Marg]

In addition, as Siney (1995) and Goode (1994) discuss, many of the
women in their studies on maternal drug use were unable to cease their
illicit drug use during pregnancy. Others described their confusion concerning their illicit drug use when they were pregnant. Similiar to
Irwin's (1995) findings, many of the mothers worried that they were
hurting their unborn children, though not intentionally. Abstaining from
illicit drug use was more complex than just saying 'no':

I became pregnant and really thought immediately that abortion ... was the only
sane thing to do at this point. He really fought me on the issue and thought that
we could quit using drugs and go out and build a picket fence and everything
would be fine. I looked at him like 'Are you nuts? Neither one of us has the capa-
bility of doing that right now.' But what a nice dream, to go back to being somewhat happy and normal again. So I let him talk me out of it. [Pat]

I didn't know what to do. I was pregnant and I was using and I didn't want to be pregnant by myself ... I didn't want to have it. So, I thought, how can I have this? I can't even be with my other child. [Mary]

I got pregnant when I was trying to clean up. I'd been trying to clean up for a year. But that's the thing. They never thought about ... the fact I had a problem ... I wasn't out there doing drugs to hurt the baby. It wasn't like, 'Oh, I think I'll go get pregnant and then I think I'll go get high and hurt this baby, so that it comes out all screwed up so everyone has to deal with my mistakes.' You know, if I wasn't prepared to deal with my mistakes I would have had an abortion ... I wouldn't have kept it. It's just hard. It's just really hard. [Karen]

Not all of the women interviewed had used drugs during their pregnancies. For those who did, the decision to continue their pregnancies was a challenge and was often stressful. Factual information about the effects of illicit drugs on maternal health was difficult to obtain. Many of the mothers were given information that greatly exaggerated the negative effects of prenatal drug use on the developing foetus, and many others received no information at all. One young Native Indian mother explained:

I didn't know nothing; I did the drugs till he was born. No one talked back then about what drugs are going to do to the baby. Nobody ever said anything to me ... I didn't know I was pregnant till I was six months pregnant, a month before I delivered. I didn't show, I even had my period ... I didn't know anything; I was on the street. [Jane]

A young mother of European heritage noted:

No one ever told me. [They'd say,] 'It's just bad for it, it'll kill the baby, and hurt the baby.' But they never told me in plain terms exactly what it did. [Karen]

As Handwerker (1994) states, physicians tend to be overly cautious in determining risk factors in pregnancy, and never remove the 'high risk' label, regardless of improvement or evidence to the contrary. Women who use illicit drugs during pregnancy are seen as being 'at risk' regardless of maternal outcomes.

After initially finding out they were pregnant, many of the women looked for prenatal care. Although there are some supportive doctors who work with women who use illicit drugs during pregnancy, many of the mothers interviewed had traumatic experiences similiar to the women Irwin (1995) interviewed in the United States. Once they were identified as illicit drug users, they were treated harshly by doctors. One mother on social assistance stated:

I went in and waited for almost three hours before I saw the doctor ... I wanted help, I needed help right. And she just dug her fingers in my ribs; I had red marks ... it was just like I was a piece of meat. It was just awful. I walked out of there and I forget what it was that she wanted. I had tears running down my eyes. And I thought, 'I'll never come back here again, no way.' And I walked out of there and I cried and I cried ... It was late – 5:30, 6:00 – before I got home. The next day, my girlfriend came home and said, 'What's wrong?' and I told her what happened ... nobody, ever, should be ... treated that way. [Ellie]

Some of the women were on methadone programs when they discovered they were pregnant. Views regarding methadone and pregnancy have shifted over the years. Currently it is suggested that methadone may benefit pregnancy by stabilizing a mother's drug use; however, infants exposed prenatally to methadone experience more severe withdrawal symptoms than infants exposed only to heroin (Institute for the Study of Drug Dependence [ISSD], 1992). In the past, women who were on legal methadone were advised by their doctors to stay on it rather than attempt withdrawal, for fear of miscarriage (Hepburn, 1993b).

Some women were told that methadone did not cross the placental barrier, so the baby would not be affected by their mother's drug use. Two long-term legal methadone patients stated:

I went on the methadone program and I wasn't affected in the way that a lot of women are today ... Of course when I went on the methadone program you were encouraged to go on ... I was told it didn't cross the placental barrier ... Since then of course they found that sometimes it does, it seems, and sometimes it doesn't, but this is what I was told. Now, ... [if] I had known that it crossed ... I likely still would have stayed on the methadone program ... Nobody wants their child born addicted ... Now, if anything, I would encourage girls not to get pregnant ... when they are on methadone ... But, life isn't that simple. It's like saying to anyone, 'Don't get pregnant.' And then, the other thing that happens ... is that women don't get their period when they are using heroin ... I'm embarrassed to tell you this. I was twenty-six weeks and I didn't know I was pregnant. Twenty-six weeks. [Linda]

There is so much misinformation ... when I found out I was pregnant, I was on methadone and the doctor of the program then was wonderful. He told me it was basically my choice of what I wanted to do. He said to me that he has a lot of experience with ... pregnant women who were addicted. He said if the women were taking care of themselves in terms of nutrition and sleep ... the babies were okay. Often they were a little less birth weight, probably, but it didn't affect intelligence and all of that. He said that alcohol and cigarettes are more dangerous than my drug. [Diane]

These mothers had few choices when they discovered that they were pregnant. Abortion was not a viable option for some of the women in the study, for prior to the discontinuation of therapeutic abortion committees in Canada abortion was a medical decision, not a woman's right (Brodie, Gavigan, & Jenson, 1992). In addition, many women who use illicit drugs cease to menstruate, so pregnancy is often not detected until after the first trimester, when abortion is not as feasible or readily available.

The information women received differed according to when and by whom they were seen during their pregnancies. Some received accurate information, but the majority did not. Therefore, pregnancy was fraught with many fears concerning outcome and possible harm to the developing foetus.

The Birth Experience

Some of the women interviewed described the negative treatment they received at the time of birth once they were identified as illicit drug users. The birth experience for most women in Western countries is situated firmly within the medical model of health, which increasingly relies on technology to monitor, predict, and confirm pregnancy and to facilitate birth (Oakley, 1986; 1992; Rothman, 1989; Saxell, 1994; Wagner, 1994). Women's subjective experience of birth is overridden by the objective knowledge of the doctor and by technological interventions (Oakley, 1992; Saxell, 1994). For many women, including the women interviewed, birth is a frightening experience, in which they have little control over their own bodies or the place and type of birth. It was not until the 1960s that home births and midwives became conditionally available to women in North America (Burtch, 1994). In Canada, midwifery is still illegal in many provinces. In B.C., it became legal in 1994; however, it was not until 1 January 1998 that midwifery services were covered by B.C. medical insurance. So the majority of women in B.C., including the women in this study, had few alternatives to the medical model of health during pregnancy, labour, and birth.

Women who use illicit drugs are considered to be 'at risk' during pregnancy and birth. However, risk assessments often have negative effects on maternal health for women (Brodie & Thompson, 1981; Handwerker, 1984; Oakley, 1992). Labelling women 'at risk' becomes problematic when women are unable to change their behaviour (Handwerker, 1984; Oakley, 1992). Women who are unable to discontinue their illicit drug use during pregnancy are perceived as failing to comply with medical advice, and this often has negative consequences for them. Moreover, female illicit drug users are often treated harshly by medical professionals, which subsequently influences their willingness to seek medical advice (Irwin, 1995). Women identified during birth as illicit drug users have been stigmatized by the medical professionals attending them at birth. Two mothers who were on social assistance at the time of birth note:

I had a PID [pelvic inflammatory disease] infection when I was pregnant. I didn't notice. I was not dilating ... fourteen hours later and I am screaming, because I had hard labour for ten or twelve hours. [They asked if there was any] reason why [I] wouldn't dilate. I, said, 'A couple of years ago I had a PID infection.' It wasn't half an hour, I was under anaesthetic and they were doing a caesarean after fourteen hours. That really blew me. It was because at first they just thought 'Oh well, it is the drugs, let them wear off. Let her suffer through it and then' ... you know, that was a trip. I mean it was pretty obvious, What was going on. As soon as they realized what was going on, sure enough, they took the baby out and I was completely infected inside. But they blamed the enlarged liver on the drugs only. Nothing to do with the infection ... of course. [Theresa]

Well, as time went on, you know, I did get down to just snorting coke and then I would go back out on the streets and fix. It was an ongoing battle trying to keep the drugs away from me. Which I wasn't able to do. And ... just before she was born, I was using the most that I ever have during the pregnancy. So, I went into labour. I was still fixing. I didn't want to go to the hospital. My water had broken and I did [go]. I had so many sores all over my body. I don't know what it was that I had, but I mean sores from head to fucking toe. I looked like a leper. I was so ill. I went into the hospital and they just ahhhh!! They were like, God! ... There was no point in even saying anything to these people. There is nothing you can do ... to justify what you have done. You can barely justify it to yourself. And there is going to be no understanding whatsoever for where you have been, what has been going on. It is like ... you are a leper. 'We don't want to touch you' ... but, then of course she was born. And it was the most painful birth I have ever had in my life ... I mean I had an epidural. I had everything ... I love having babies. I mean, all my children up until then, I really enjoyed their births. This was so damn painful, this was 'Give me anything ... to stop the pain.' I didn't know ... and I thought these were the stories that my mother had told me about birth. [Pat]

For many women ceasing illicit drug use during pregnancy is a challenge, and many are unsuccessful. But continued drug use is not in itself irresponsible; as Oakley (1992) noted in relation to smoking, it is a way for many women to deal with the stresses of their lives and their domestic environments, and to continue caring for their families. Morgan and Joe (1997), Goode (1994), and Taylor (1993) discovered that women often tend to use illicit drugs to cope with family life and to gain a sense of control over their situation. There is a wide range of responses and motivations for continued use of illicit drugs, including positive motivations and coping motivations. Using illicit drugs to cope with social stresses does not indicate lack of agency. Rather, it suggests that women actively search for ways to enhance or alter their realities. The choice of an illicit drug over other possibilities may be shaped by social, political, cultural, and economic variables.

Parenting and Guilt

Like other mothers who use illicit drugs and have participated in sociological studies (see Colten, 1980, 1982; Irwin, 1995; Kearny et al., 1994; Rosenbaum, 1981; Taylor, 1993), all of the women interviewed in this study conformed to the ideology of motherhood in their acceptance of their role as the primary caregivers for their children, and in the subsequent guilt they experienced as mothers who use illicit drugs. Many discussed their fear of losing their children either temporarily or permanently through child apprehension by the Ministry of Social Services. Many discussed the guilt they experienced as mothers who used illicit drugs. For those who used illicit drugs during pregnancy, and for women whose children were occasionally exposed to illicit activities, the guilt experienced was immense. Overwhelmingly, regardless of race and class, the women interviewed expressed guilt concerning their illicit drug use and its negative impact on children, friends, and family:

I suffered tremendous guilt. I know that it stopped me ... from doing lots of things in my life ... I just felt crippled. I never knew what that word [guilt] meant until I was forty years old ... It is my biggest enemy and my constant companion, is guilt. [Judy]

I think I feel guilty ... because of what I put my parents through and what I put my daughter through and all that stuff. [Diane]

The mothers interviewed viewed themselves as responsible for both their own behaviour and the behaviour of their partners:

Oh yeah, I felt the guilt. Because obviously I was poisoning them inside [during pregnancy], and being a mother I was responsible; I should have been responsible. Even to the point where I should have been responsible for his behaviour. Which was really stupid. I ended up feeling responsible for everything. And lost of course. It was a losing battle by that time. [Donna]

I felt responsible for everything that was going on in my life. [Pat]

Adhering to familial ideology, the women carried the total burden of parenting. This is not to imply that understanding the role of mothering that prevails in Western culture would have allowed them to escape their guilt and feeling of sole responsibility of their children. Many of them were fully aware of the sexism that structured their lives. What is most significant is their almost universal experience of men as absent caregivers and of society's failure to offer support. It is from this place that the women interviewed took on the traditional role of caregiver. The guilt they experienced in relation to their children was all the more painful because they saw no viable options, especially when they were poor:

You know, when the kids were not going to school, they were driving with me. That is all they did, was travel looking for dope. And I feel terrible about that. God, I feel guilty about that ... As a mother, you are going to feel guilty about using dope. I mean ... you are constantly getting it from society. [Theresa]

It might have been easy for me if I had given her up from the moment she was born. Then you don't have so many memories, regrets, and guilt. [Pat]

As the one mother noted above, when women fail to feel guilt about their illicit drug use, society is always ready to remind them that such drug use is not consistent with good mothering.

Adhering to the ideology of mothering that prevails in Western culture, many of the mothers expressed their regret that their children were exposed to their activities as illicit drug users; they all felt personally responsible for this exposure, even though the criminalization of drugs plays a large part in shaping illicit drug use. In fact, the majority of the mothers were in favour of decriminalization and were aware of the negative implications of the criminalization of drugs and of social attitudes. Still, when discussing their children, they took full responsibility for every aspect of their care. They hoped to shield them from harm, and when that was not successful they felt tremendous guilt about their lifestyles.

Many of the women expressed their concern about raising children in Canadian society. They discussed the importance of educating their children about illicit drug use, and about the economic, social, and political structure of Canadian society that perpetuates stereotypes about illicit drug use. Some spoke about their fears:

I had a lot of anger, but for my children, too. I'm really worried about them, too. Not really worried about using, because I plan to educate them well, but just growing up in our society. [Morgan]

The only thing I hated about my parents is they were hypocrites: 'Do as I say, not as I do.' And I hated that. And I'm going to try my best ... I'm not saying I'm going to be perfect, but I'm going to try to be honest with her, because how [else] can I expect her to be honest with me? ... I want her to be able to talk to me, but how can she talk to me if I can't talk to her? A lot of ... things to learn. I want to go to parenting classes. [Karen]

And this is one of the reasons I really want to keep ... the anti-prohibition movement going, because I don't want my daughter going through what I did. I don't want anybody's kid going through what I had to go through. [Theresa]

The mothers educated their children, and strove for shifts in social attitudes surrounding illicit drug use. Maintaining open communication with their children appeared to be important to the mothers, especially as their children reached adulthood. One long-term legal methadone patient stated:

Yes, when she was old enough ... I knew that there would become a time and to ... simply ignore the whole thing would be very bad on my part. So I knew at one point we would have a good talk. Because she knew ... she was in her young teens, thirteen, I think it was. I sat her down ... and talked with her about the methadone. She was like, 'I know, Mom' ... probably I could have talked to her a couple of years earlier and didn't even realize it. But she knew, you know. But she respected that I was honest with her. I think that was important ... You know, [it] ... would have been horribly wrong on my part to try to fool her. [Evelyn]

Many of the mothers, both single parents and mothers who had a supportive partner, hoped and strove for changes in drug legislation and social attitudes, and educated their children about illicit drug use as they reached adulthood.

Conclusion

Rather than exploring the many constraints that women, and especially mothers, experience in relation to their roles as caretakers, women are blamed for failing to cease their illicit (and licit) drug use. Subsequently, women blame themselves. Rather than examining the social context of women's lives, health professionals question whether a mother exhibits sufficient responsibility towards her developing foetus, and whether she has followed medical advice. Consequently, maternal health can be seen as a matter of individual choice rather than a result of the mother's social environment. Mothers are blamed for the outcomes of their pregnancies, and infants labelled with neonatal abstinence syndrome (NAS) are subject to further medical surveillance.

3

Neonatal Abstinence Syndrome (NAS): Sunny Hill Hospital for Children

Of the children of the twenty-eight mothers interviewed for this study, fourteen of their children had been diagnosed with neonatal abstinence syndrome (NAS). Of these fourteen children, ten were in-patients at the NAS program at Sunny Hill Hospital for Children in Vancouver, B.C. All of the mothers were on social assistance when their children were transferred to the in-patient NAS program at Sunny Hill, and seven of the ten children were eventually permanently apprehended by the Ministry of Social Services (see table 3.1).

The ideologies surrounding mothering, family, and illicit drugs often inform medical decision making regarding the care of infants. Both historically and in contemporary society, medical professionals have instructed women about how to behave during pregnancy and child rearing (Arnup, 1994; Davin, 1978; King, 1989; Mitchinson, 1988). Specifically, certain activities have been forbidden. Rarely are the doctors' instructions, advice, assessment, and treatment challenged. And rarely are doctors perceived as hazardous to health[1] (Rothman, 1989). The treatment of infants labelled 'at risk' for NAS at Sunny Hill Hospital demonstrates how mothers are controlled and punished outside of the criminal law.

The Sunny Hill Hospital NAS Program

Until 1983, there was no specialized program for infants experiencing neonatal abstinence syndrome (NAS) in British Columbia. The label NAS was first used by Finnegan (1979) to describe symptoms of infant withdrawal and guidelines for care. Infants in B.C. diagnosed with NAS were treated individually by doctors at hospitals, or as out-patients, throughout

TABLE 3.1
Biographical data on mothers of infants sent to Sunny Hill in-patient program

Total Mothers: 8	Total Children: 10			
	N	%	N	%
On social assistance when infant was transferred to NAS in-patient program	8	100		
European Heritage	4	50	5	50
African American	1	12	1	10
Native Indian	3	37	4	40

the province. The women in this study who gave birth prior to 1983 had a wide range of experiences that differed from those of women who gave birth in or after 1983. For the women who gave birth prior to 1983, the label NAS was not used by medical professionals, and treatment differed, depending on the doctor they chose.

Not all infants exposed to maternal drug use experience NAS. Research has found no correlation between severity of withdrawal symptoms and length and quantity of maternal drug use (Fricker & Segal, 1978; Hepburn, 1993a). What is most significant about the labelling and treatment of NAS is the perception of the mothers interviewed and the care of the infants. The mothers discussed the changes that occurred in B.C. once Sunny Hill Hospital for Children developed its NAS program in 1983.

Sunny Hill Hospital for Children, a fifty-five-bed paediatric rehabilitation centre in Vancouver, has the only NAS program in the province of British Columbia. The founding physician of the program was its medical director until 1992. Between 360 and 372 infants were treated as NAS in-patients over the first ten years of the program (Sunny Hill Hospital Tertiary Task Force, 1993, p. 6).

In March 1992 a formal task force came together from the B.C. Ministry of Health to evaluate the care provided by the NAS program at Sunny Hill Hospital; the Ministry of Health declared that the NAS program was both 'atypical' and 'expensive' (Sunny Hill Tertiary Task Force, 1993). Dr Susan Albersheim notes that the NAS in-patient program at Sunny Hill Hospital was no different from other programs across Canada (Sunny Hill Tertiary Task Force, 1993). But this is a rather general statement that overlooks the physical environment, the length of stay, and the physical care of the infants in the program. In 1992, a new medical director of the NAS program was appointed. By 1994, small but significant changes had occurred. Because it is too early to assess the current program at Sunny Hill, this study is concerned with the NAS program prior to 1993.

Denial and Lies

The founding director of the Sunny Hill NAS program explained that he began his work with infants prenatally exposed to drugs prior to 1983, at Vancouver General Hospital (VGH):

I was impressed by the fact that the mothers themselves suffer what addicts do anyway, they are despised, looked down upon, and so on, by the rest of society. [1][2]

He was especially concerned with the suffering infants experienced due to their mothers' maternal drug use:

I realized that nobody knew how to treat them, and not too many people cared very much. So that is how I got into it ... I came back from Harvard training in '57. So from '57 on I was in the nurseries at VGH, and than I became head of the nursery here. So ... these women, I didn't treat them like savages, but more than that, I really cared about the babies. [1]

When VGH moved its paediatrics and maternity departments to Grace Hospital and Shaughnessy Hospital, the founding director continued his work at these hospitals until the NAS program was created at Sunny Hill Hospital in 1983. Although the program he set up was primarily concerned with the medical treatment of infants experiencing NAS, parents were also affected by their infants' stay in hospital. Although the director hoped to establish a program that would better meet the needs of the infants, and thus the parents, often his assumptions about both the infants and their parents became embedded in the policy governing the medical care of these infants. For the mothers interviewed, the policy at the Sunny Hill Hospital NAS program was viewed as problematic and threatening.

It is well documented that women are reluctant to go for medical care if they fear child apprehension and personal stigmatization (Chavkin, Allen, & Oberman, 1991; Gómez, 1994; Maher, 1992; Humphries et al., 1992; Siney, 1994). Some of the mothers interviewed acknowledged that they avoided contact with medical professionals while pregnant. The mothers' fear of approaching the medical community for help during pregnancy is further complicated by the medical professionals' belief that women lie or are in denial about their drug use (Robins & Mills, 1993; Stone, Salerno, Green, & Zelson, 1971; Williams & Bruce, 1994). As the founding director of the NAS program observed,

> There is enough variation [in] what mothers take and seldom they tell the truth anyway. They may intentionally tell a lie; many of them tell lies. And they block out certain things. [1]

Lauridsen-Hoegh, the NAS program coordinator, claims that the parents of the infants treated in their program are extremely manipulative (1991, p. 15). Given the founding director's and program coordinator's frame of reference that mothers fail to tell the truth, and their position, it would be difficult for some birth parents to form therapeutic relationships with the medical staff at the program. Rather than claiming that mothers who use drugs manipulate and lie, and assuming that mothers take more drugs than they admit to, one could more usefully analyse the environment of mistrust that exists between the mothers and the medical community.

Infants Labelled NAS

Infants were usually referred from St Paul's Hospital and B.C. Children's Hospital to Sunny Hill Hospital's NAS program. Nurses, social workers, and physicians identified infants who were at risk for NAS, and the founding director of the NAS program approved their transfer to Sunny Hill. Two small residential rooms had been set aside for infants labelled NAS at Sunny Hill; the rest of the hospital cares for children with acute and terminal illnesses. As mentioned earlier, fourteen children were diagnosed with NAS. Of these children, ten were treated as in-patients at Sunny Hill. The other four infants who were not treated as in-patients included one child diagnosed with NAS at a few months of age, and a set of twins diagnosed at the age of four. These three had only been treated as out-patients at Sunny Hill. One other infant was born and treated for NAS in Ontario.
According to the mothers interviewed, not all of the fourteen children showed clinical signs of NAS. Nevertheless, ten of them were kept in special care nurseries at B.C. Children's Hospital and St Paul's Hospital, and later referred to the in-patient NAS program at Sunny Hill. Clinical manifestations of withdrawal are separated into two categories at Sunny Hill.

Life-threatening manifestations include explosive diarrhoea; water depletion, shock, projectile or continuous vomiting, and convulsions. Nonthreatening manifestations include tremors; hyperreflexia; exaggerated Moro response; excessive sweating; fever without apparent cause; sneezing and snuffles; hiccups; hyperactivity; denuding knees elbows and nose; excessive crying; feeding, sucking, and swallowing dysfunctions; lethargy; floppiness; arching of the back; intolerance of handling; skin mottling; high-pitched crying; distressing insomnia; unexplained failure to gain weight; light intolerance; and coughing (Sunny Hill Hospital for Children, 1992a).

However, these symptoms may not appear in infants exposed prenatally to drugs. Withdrawal symptoms are not predictable or inevitable, and they range widely. The Sunny Hill Hospital Tertiary Task Force stated that infants (360–72 infants during the first ten years) were referred to Sunny Hill if the referring hospital felt that the infant was in need of specialized treatment for NAS; if the social environment of the parents was complex and could delay discharge; if there was a past history of drug use by the mother; if there was high risk due to the ethnicity of the mother; and if there was a lack of foster-care placement after an infant has been apprehended from the parents (Sunny Hill Hospital Tertiary Task Force, 1993, pp. 3, 4). Consequently, many infants who were not exhibiting NAS symptoms are sent to the NAS in-patient program at Sunny Hill Hospital. Unfortunately, all infants referred to the program were treated for NAS, regardless of their lack of symptoms.

Many of the mothers interviewed appeared confused about why their children were kept in special care nurseries and later transferred to Sunny Hill:

My daughter was born at seven pounds. That is not bad, yet where was she ... ICU [intensive care unit]. [There was] no reason for any of this ... They kept trying to tell me that she was wired and crying ... well if you had something stuck in your goddamn head and you can't move, wouldn't you be cranky and crying too? Yeah, and I mean it was two weeks before I could even touch the baby ... They kept her in for a month [at St Paul's]. And I was really frightened at the time that I was going to lose her, that this was just ... a waiting game. [Theresa]

Another mother did not see her infant for ten days after his birth:

I didn't see him for the first ten days, but they told me he didn't show too much of any signs. [Lori]

She had been told by the Ministry of Social Services that unless she went into a drug treatment centre her infant would not be returned to her, even though the infant did not appear to be showing serious symptoms. Another mother whose infant had no obvious symptoms of NAS stated:

He [the director] has one general prescription for all babies; he doesn't look at the degrees of damage done to them. [Greta]

Mothers were also frightened by the setting of the program and the acute patients treated there. Many of the children residing at the hospital are mentally and physically handicapped. Mothers interviewed feared that their children admitted for NAS were perceived as being as ill as the other children admitted to Sunny Hill. Rarely was it explained that NAS is transitory. One mother noted her husband's reaction to Sunny Hill:

It scared my husband. He had no idea about this stuff, and we would go in, and he would call them broken children, he didn't understand the ones that are slightly retarded or physically broken and it scared the hell out of him. [Donna]

Aside from the intimidating hospital setting, parents were also troubled by the environment allocated specifically to NAS infants, the medical treatment, the close alliance with social services, their infants' long confinement in hospital, and the surveillance of their care of their infants.

In-patient Stay

Infants transferred to Sunny Hill were kept in two tiny darkened rooms with no intercom system and no special care nursery medical equipment. It is interesting to note that infants who had been identified as requiring specialized care were left in an isolated room where there was no communication system set up for the nurses to contact outside help. The bleak rooms could each accommodate six NAS infants. Black-out curtains surrounded each crib, protecting the child from light and noise, and night lights were used for observation of the children (Lauridsen-Hoegh, 1991, p. 14). The infants lay in large cribs all day and night. Sound and touch was limited. Mothers and medical staff were not allowed to touch the children, except briefly at feeding, bathing, and changing times. Infants were not cuddled, rocked, spoken to, or brought outside the room into the light for fear that they would become overstimulated. Mothers could speak to their children only occasionally, in hushed voices. Additional auditory stimulation was guarded against. Infants were placed in this environment of sensory deprivation immediately after staying in special care nurseries, which generally have lights on twenty-four hours a day, lots of noise, and nurses, doctors, parents, and other family members visiting.

At Sunny Hill it was believed that infants labelled NAS need a low-stimulation environment to reduce the severity of withdrawal (Lauridsen-Hoegh, 1991). Therefore, the two rooms set aside for NAS in-patients were designed for maximum sensory deprivation. Infants are kept within the black-out curtains until 'symptomatically justified' (Lauridsen-Hoegh, 1991, p. 14). When the past director of the NAS program was asked about the average length of time infants stayed in the darkened rooms, he stated:

The average is not too meaningful, there is such a wide, wide variation. There are probably very few who went home in less than three weeks and some of them were here for six months. [1]

However, to the mothers interviewed, the length of time (up to six months) their infants resided in the darkened rooms was significant:

She was born at Grace [Hospital], but they moved her within a couple of weeks to Sunny Hill ... she was there for five months. [Pat]

Two months in the darkened room ... I put her two months behind for being in Sunny Hill because she was deprived of contact. [Donna]

She spent about two weeks at Grace Hospital. Then they found out she had withdrawal ... so they took her to Sunny Hill and put her in the dark room. She stayed there until she was about five months old. [Grace]

In contrast, the majority of infants labelled NAS in other programs in Scotland and England return home within three to fourteen days (Hepburn, 1993a; Institute for the Study of Drug Dependence [ISDD], 1992; Siney, 1994). Infants perceived as no longer needing the low stimulation at Sunny Hill were sent home within a few days of coming out of the isolated, darkened room. However, parents believed that the time their infants spent in these rooms may have contributed to poor development and later adjustment problems.

When the founding director was asked if the mothers were allowed to touch their infants when they were in these darkened rooms, he stated:

There is no real allowable amount of stimulation. It's a matter of having to handle them to change their diaper and to feed them ... but in the ordinary course of rocking the baby, you know that sort of thing seems to add to their stimulation. Occasionally a baby will be soothed by being rocked but ... usually chemically dependent mothers do not have what many other mothers have, that sensitivity to what the baby will tolerate. So instead of being soothing, they will handle the baby and shake the baby and so on ... they are devoted, but whatever it is that guides other mothers, they don't seem to have ... The nurses were aware of that, and at the same time they were torn, torn by the knowledge that these are the mothers, they want to handle their babies. [1]

The ideology of mothering shapes the medical practice at Sunny Hill. Mothering is a social construct rather than a biological imperative (Arnup, 1994; Glenn, 1994). But by portraying mothering as natural, the 'medical expert' can claim that certain women, that is, women who use illicit drugs, do not possess these inherent qualities. Although the nurses found the medical protocol at the NAS program contrary to their own knowledge about mothering and comforting infants, they were instructed that the mothers of NAS infants lacked the maternal knowledge (instinct) to comfort their own children. The nurses also adopted the expert's opinion on mothering, which denied their own knowledge. Therefore the medical protocol regulating and limiting stimulation, including touch, was enforced by the nurses and medical staff, even though there is no medical evidence supporting lack of touch in the literature on NAS.

In contrast to the program at Sunny Hill, NAS programs in England and Scotland encourage both touch and the active participation of mothers, by having the infants remain with their mothers after birth (Siney, 1994; Hepburn, 1993a, 1993b). Only a small percentage of infants whose symptoms are severe (which is rare) require more specialized care (Siney, 1994; Hepburn, 1993a, 1993b). These infants are not shielded from light, noise, or touch (Siney, 1994; Hepburn, 1993a, 1993b).

Other NAS programs in the United States discuss the need to shield infants from direct bright lights (Greider, 1995); however, natural outdoor light and bedside lights are acceptable (Lowe & Ehrhard-Wingard, 1994). Some programs have incorporated infant massage into their treatment regimen, and parents are encouraged and instructed to touch and massage their infants (Lowe & Ehrhard-Wingard, 1994). Winnicott states: 'It is the physical holding of the physical frame that provides the psychology that can be good or bad ... Babies do not remember being held well –

what they remember is the traumatic experience of not being held well enough.' (1987, p. 62, 63)

Winnicott (1987) suggests that infants cannot exist alone and are part of a relationship. Many health professionals that care for infants recognize that 'the parent–infant pair must be cared for as a unit' (Brazelton & Cramer, 1990, p. xv). Parent–infant interaction is a neccessary component of infant development (Brazelton & Cramer, 1990; Winnicott, 1987). Parent–infant interaction and behaviour signal and determine responses, 'one member acting on and shaping the other, but also acted upon and shaped *by* the other' (Brazelton & Cramer, 1990, p. 97). In addition, stimulation is necessary to the maturation of sensory organs (p. 27).

Outside of Sunny Hill, it is believed that human contact is essential in the care of infants labelled NAS, and that a home-like environment should be incorporated into NAS programs (Lowe & Ehrhard-Wingard, 1994). Some doctors suggest that loud, startling noises should be avoided (Lowe & Ehrhard-Wingard, 1994). Others have no policy on noise; therefore, the infants would be exposed to the same level of noise any other infant would be after birth (Siney, 1994; Hepburn, 1993a, 1993b).

Isolating infants in darkened rooms for long periods of time is unique to the NAS in-patient program at Sunny Hill. Most programs recognize that infant withdrawal varies in length. Generally the physiological effects of withdrawal last for three to fourteen days. It is rare for it to last more than two weeks (ISDD, 1992). Any other negative effects experienced by infants may be due to prematurity or health problems unrelated to their mothers' drug use. There is no medical reason to keep them in isolation and darkness for such long periods of time, especially given the availability of various medications that may alleviate withdrawal symptoms.

The regulations and protocol for infants' care at Sunny Hill's NAS in-patient program concerned the mothers:

They let me hold them for a couple of minutes but they didn't want them stimulated. [Liz]

We would go down, and have to put on these gowns and these gloves. I always refused to put on the gloves. White gloves and go in and not make any noise [Donna]

Well there was two of them in the room, but you had to keep it quiet ... They had the curtains closed and you had to be quiet. [Jill]

Mothers expressed concern that the treatment their infants received at

Sunny Hill was damaging to their infants' health. One Native mother was concerned that her child was never encouraged to sit up or crawl because he was confined to his crib:

He just lay there, and he got fatter and fatter. He's not moving and they wouldn't let him go crawling. [Jill]

Other mothers were concerned with the lack of bonding and the institutional setting, which appeared cold and uncaring:

And one of the things, too, is you're breaking the bonding, and then the mother may never bond. The baby may never bond. [Janet]

They are fed on a clock basis, and if they cry, they just go and poke a soother in their mouth ... Just a soother. They will pop it in and turn them over and cover them up again and that is it. It was cold in there too ... Yes, they got the big cribs for them. You are not supposed to bother them. I took the responsibility of feeding periods which was just limited to us for half an hour and they kept the room dark and cold. I guess she had to sweat it out. Half an hour, we were gone ... When your time was up, it was like you were in jail or something. You know, you just walked in and you are supposed to be really ... like a matron or something. Pick up the baby, feed her, change her, put her back to bed and that was it. And they never had the babies warm or anything. It was always one little blanket to sleep with. I found it really ... awful the way that they looked after the babies. [Grace]

Infants were fed every three hours. They were said to have 'hypermetabolic demands,' where their systems are in 'fast forward,' and to require structured feedings until steady weight gains were achieved according to established growth curves (Lauridsen-Hoegh, 1991, p. 15). This protocol to measure progress through weight gain directly affected the mothers and infants:

They wanted him to be fed in twenty minutes. So what if it took an hour? It was my business. [Greta]

Infants were also given a high-calorie formula when they were on medication. Progress was noted on a flow sheet. About 30 to 50 per cent of the infants received a paediatric opium solution, similar to paregoric but free of camphor and other toxins, and with the alcohol concentration reduced (Lauridsen-Hoegh, 1991, p. 14). However, mothers expressed concern that infants who had not been exposed maternally to opiate derivatives were also prescribed paregoric:

When we went in the room, it was dark at first, she was on opium and stuff, and I was using cocaine and I thought, 'This is stupid ... why put them on opium when it was cocaine?' And they said, 'It makes their coming into the world easier' ... I think it slowed her in some ways. [Donna]

Parents' expressed concerns about the medical treatment of their infants with opiates were not recognized as valid. The founding director stated:

A chemically dependent person, male or female, does not want anybody saying ... they should be doing this or that. So if I decide to put a baby on opium, they may feel 'Well, this guy's not going to do that without my permission.' So there was that kind of resentment; they just didn't want to be controlled. [1]

Instead of recognizing that parents had legitimate concerns related to their infants' care and the medical treatment they received in the program, medical staff perceived parents as not wishing to be controlled.

Sunny Hill Hospital also notes that NAS infants have poor sucking responses, and feeding, sucking, and swallowing dysfunctions (Sunny Hill Hospital, 1992a). However, they do not raise the question of how forced feeding and bottle-feeding, as opposed to breast-feeding, affects infants' sucking response. In the film *Saint Segal,* a nurse is shown attempting to feed one of the infants in the in-patient NAS program. Contrary to program policy, she is roughly jiggling the infant and bottle in her attempt to get the maximum amount of milk into the infant. Babies need time to breathe in between sucking, and differ in their sucking and eating habits. Forcing them to eat within a prescribed time limit may contribute to the running of an efficient hospital program, but rigid routines fail to address the individual needs of each infant.

Not all of the mothers believed that their infants were experiencing NAS, and many questioned the inevitability of NAS symptoms as expressed by medical professionals. Mothers noted that their infants did not always follow the pattern of NAS predicted by the medical professionals at Sunny Hill. They felt that their infants were not as 'ill' or 'unattached' as the medical professionals claimed:

Yeah, they try to act like just everything was because of the drugs. And I know differently. Some of those [symptoms] were just baby things ... he [the director] kept trying to act like 'Any day now it's gonna happen; you are going to see these symptoms.' [Greta]

The founding director believed that infants experiencing NAS were unable to bond with their caregivers. Isolating infants in small darkened rooms and depriving them of touch, sound, and light did not interfere with bonding because the physiological sequelae of withdrawal made it impossible for the infants to bond:

Now in a state of withdrawal they are in no mood to bond or anything, and being touched upsets them. And ... I don't think it is an exaggeration to liken that situation to somebody who pays a lot of money to go to a symphony and then comes down with a migraine headache. And that's what's frightening about these babies; they are in no position to be receptive to ... nurturing [1].

He also noted that:

These kids go through a social experience, which when they are old enough, I'm thinking weeks, months ... they learn to socialize in terms of making eye contact, in terms of capturing a person's attention and being affected if the other person looks away ... it's a social skill which to many people would be evidence that this kid is bonding. But he's not. It's a form of manipulation. And ... of course street life is like this. People watch the eyes of their victims. There's a lot of nonverbal communication in most of us. But street people go by it. And these babies aren't street people, but a person can have no loyalties to any friend, no sense of social values and anything like that, but can have a tremendous bedside manner, be really engaging. Of course that makes that person more dangerous ... These babies can develop a social skill that ... makes them very responsive to whoever [is] there, and yet they may have passed the time ... when they couldn't possibly be attached to anybody ... there comes an age when that bonding process doesn't seem to happen, and in a normal child it is somewhere around nine months of age. [1]

The director confused his own ill-informed image of poverty and street life with the effects of maternal drug use. The ideological assumptions that the director held about poor people, illicit drug use, and mothers were camouflaged as medical expertise.

Infants exposed to cocaine prenatally are often said to be recognizable by their behavioural differences and their 'unreachableness' in interpersonal relationships; however, Robins and Mills note that they are no different from other children from economically and socially deprived backgrounds (1993, p. 29). Furthermore, Hawley and Disney (1992) point out that children who remain with their biological mothers are securely attached.

The mothers interviewed were especially sensitive to the fact that their infants had bonded to them, contrary to the medical information they had received at Sunny Hill, and they expressed their concerns at length during the interviews:

He had to eat his words, because my son was so bonded to me that he just stared at me whenever he heard my voice. And the director said, 'I've never seen a baby that attached, that much attachment in a baby that small.' Because he would just stare into my eyes like nobody else existed. He said he probably wouldn't be able to look at me and they have trouble bonding and all this stuff. [Greta]

Yeah, I remember them saying 'Your son is not going to know you,' and all that. And I thought, 'Not my son, he's going to know his mum.' [Ellie]

The way they told me about C., that she couldn't make friends with people and she wouldn't be cuddly, and she wouldn't be warm. That she would always be ... at arm's length with everybody. But, I found it really different once I started to go there. Because she started to be really waiting for us, it seemed. All what they said about her was so different. I was expecting to find a very hard child to even hold, but she was waiting all the time we would come. She would be [lying] there with her eyes open and she knew that we were there for her. I think that is what gave her the boost to fight all the odds against her. [Grace]

Some mothers thought that the way they were instructed to treat their infants shaped their infants' responses to them:

My friend's kid is a spoiled little brat and it has nothing to do with dope. It's the way we react to what they say. The rules that they give you, you are all paranoid about them, and you react really to what they tell you to expect ... I expected it [that her daughter would not bond] because she wasn't home. And that's what I got. And I was in the hospital because of my heart operation; I was gone for three months. And when I got home, she was 'I'm papa's baby,' you know. And she didn't want nothing to do with me, but of course, at first I blamed that on the dope, and then when I saw the way she was with my husband, then I said, 'This is just because [of] how I am with her.' And I've been home nine months now. It took maybe three months before she would put her hands up to me ... But ... I couldn't see that I was treating her differently until I saw how my husband was treating her when I got home, and how she was with him ... And I always said, 'Here I finally have a baby and I'm straight and she's not huggy, she doesn't want me she just wants to take off.' And that really wasn't the way she was at all. That was the way I was with her. [Donna]

The mothers felt strongly that the information they received from Sunny Hill about their children not bonding was incorrect. In fact, Sunny Hill's medical practice and information on infant attachment hindered bonding, thus creating a problem where one need not exist.

Although the founding director insists that it is the withdrawal from maternal drug use that impedes bonding, he concedes that the hospital setting also contributes to the lack of bonding:

Bonding has to be with one person, or a constant with two parents, or two guardians or whatever. With the shift system here, and very different ways that different people handle a baby, how they hold them and so on, their voices ... in a hospital setting anyway, there is no bonding. [1]

But no attempt was made until recently to change the hospital setting or to create alternatives outside of Sunny Hill. Although the founding director told me he was concerned that the hospital setting contributed to a lack of infant bonding, he never expressed these concerns to the mothers. All they were told was that their infants would not bond due to maternal drug use and the negative effects of NAS.

The majority of the mothers interviewed felt that they were not given guidelines or offered support through participation in a parents' program that might ensure that their infants were returned to them. This lack of guidelines created tension, for the mothers had no idea what was expected of them and decisions about their infants' care and discharge appeared arbitrary. One mother stated that she was given no information about how to care for her baby. However, she stated:

I'm sure if I asked them something, they would have told me. [Liz]

Given the newness of the situation, and the medicalized environment, it would have been more appropriate to give information and guidelines for infant discharge to all of the mothers upon arrival, rather than providing follow-up instructions at discharge time. As one mother stated:

They never have guidelines. It is always this open-ended stuff that it is just playing dangle, dangle with you over every fucking issue ... In the first place, they pretty much ignored me. It was like I almost wasn't there. I had trouble ... even asking directions. It was like ... I do have a right to be here, you know. And it happened every single time I came. It was like ...' [which] child is yours? Who are you?' It didn't matter how long you came, they still acted like they didn't know who the fuck you were, or what you were trying to do. [Pat]

It was important that mothers visit their infants, for visits were recorded on the infants' flow sheets and could have some influence on whether their infants would be allowed to come home. Good mothering was measured by how often a mother visited her infant, regardless of other factors that may have rendered visiting impossible. Sometimes, the nurses' surveillance of parents was beneficial to them. As one mother stated:

The nurses were great; they kept track of every time I came up to feed him. They were one of the reasons that I got him. Because they had written such good reports. 'Oh she was very good with the baby today.' They marked everything down ... in my favour. [Greta]

However, many mothers reported that they were very uncomfortable with the nurse's presence when visiting at Sunny Hill:

I found it really difficult ... because it made it seem like you were going into a prison to visit them ... You had to ... just watch how you conducted yourself. Like even looking at the baby or saying hello to it or you know ... putting your hand in the crib made you feel that you were doing something really awful. Like if you said hello to it. If the nurse was there, you couldn't, because it seemed like she was in there just to see what you were doing. And I really felt for those babies. [Grace]

They really hovered around me, like whenever I went into her room and held her or changed her or whatever, it was like all this constant hovering around by people who were trying to pretend, like they were not overseeing the situation. But [they] were. [It] made it so uncomfortable that it was ... really hard ... to stay for very long. [Pat]

The NAS program coordinator explains that, during an infant's stay at Sunny Hill, doctors rely on the 'observation and impressions related to them by the nurses' (Lauridsen-Hoegh, 1991, p. 14) for the clinical management of the infants. Unlike mothers in the Glasgow and Liverpool programs (Siney, 1994, 1995; Hepburn, 1993a), mothers were not trusted to record their own attendance and their own perceptions of their infant's health at Sunny Hill.

The institutional setting and surveillance of the mothers at Sunny Hill intimidated mothers. Mothers who opposed the prescribed medical treatment for their infants were perceived as non-compliant. Furthermore, for many mothers poverty impeded their ability to visit their infants at Sunny Hill. Many were denied bus passes by the Ministry of Social Services, and many had other children at home, which made visiting problematic. Until recently, there was no room set aside for the mothers at Sunny Hill; therefore, they had to wait in the cafeteria between feedings.

One of the powerful aspects of the ideology of mothering is that it keeps mothers in their place. There are no avenues within Sunny Hill for mothers to complain about medical protocol. Nor are there other avenues for mothers to present economic and social problems that shape mothering and attendance at Sunny Hill. Often mothering is judged on external behaviour that adheres to the ideology of mothering, which views mothers as inherently giving, pure, sacrificing, and selfless (Gupta, 1995; Thurer, 1994). Few of the mothers at Sunny Hill were able to fit into the confines of this ideology. One Native Indian mother described her difficulty in visiting both of her sons, one in Sunny Hill, the other in foster care:

We didn't have no bus fare or nothing. I had to walk to the hospital ... and Sunny Hill was over at Slocan and 20th, and J. was at Williams and Nanaimo ... It was a long walk. And you go home and sleep and next day you try to go again. It was awful. [Jill]

Another Native Indian mother, in a similar situation, says:

I went all the way to Jericho Beach to go see D., Sunny Hill to see C., and I had to phone ahead and tell them that I was coming for C. Sometimes, there was a park, Renfrew Park, I would wait around there for the next feeding, so I was there for two feedings. Then I would come home and look after [the rest of my] family. [Grace]

Long-Term NAS Problems

The Sunny Hill NAS program lists the following potential long-term NAS problems: impaired growth rate/stunting, poor movement and coordination, abnormal muscle tone, delayed speech, impaired hearing, disturbed behaviour, hyperactivity, sleep disturbances, brief attention span, learning disorders, aggressiveness, poor self-confidence, bursts of uncontrollable temper, difficulty in making and keeping friends, and defective communication skills (Sunny Hill Hospital for Children, 1992c). Many of these long-term symptoms are subjective and unsubstantiated. Nevertheless, medical policy is often constructed according to the prevailing ideology concerning illicit drugs. Illicit drugs are perceived as inherently dangerous. Infants exposed to illicit drugs are thought to suffer from the long-term problems listed above. In addition, mothers who expose their developing foetuses to the 'danger' of illicit drugs are perceived as failing to be mothers (Rosenbaum, Murphy, Irwin, & Watson, 1990).

Moreover, the ideologies surrounding both illicit drug use and mothering shape medical assumptions and policy. The past director of the Sunny Hill NAS program states:

For the chemical[ly] dependent children they don't have a sense of security that comes through attachment, they don't have a sense of loyalty to friends or elders. They don't have appreciation, or at least a motivation, to fit into social values in general. And lacking ... in a sense of security, they tend to be very aggressive and scared. [1]

The incidence of behavioural problems associated with children prenatally exposed to illicit drugs has not been substantiated. Critics state that it is not possible yet to determine behavioural problems associated with maternal drug use (Hepburn, 1993a, 1993b; Mayes, Granger, Bornstein, & Zuckerman, 1992), for studies do not distinguish among exposure to other drugs, genetic liabilities, and prenatal liabilities (Hepburn, 1993a, 1993b; Robins & Mills, 1993, p. 18). Furthermore, there is no scientific evidence that infants exposed prenatally to illicit drugs lack loyalty or a sense of social values.

For parents of the infants in the NAS program, information about their infants' development was not available except from the director and nurses. Therefore, the director's medical protocols and his underlying assumptions for establishing these protocols are important to note, especially when they were not based on medical evidence. Much of the medical treatment of the infants in program at Sunny Hill was based on 'hunches,' which in turn were based on ideological assumptions.

Social Services and Sunny Hill

The Sunny Hill program worked closely with the Ministry of Social Services. The founding director of the NAS program states:

When we started up here we developed a much closer relationship to the social workers ... not right away, but that developed to the point where we were really one with them, very close, so that we entered into the placement of the child whether it was birth mother or foster mom. [1]

However, the Native Indian community in the Lower Mainland was concerned that infants had been referred to Sunny Hill Hospital '*only* for social and economic reasons, and the effect of this was to place the infant at increased risk of apprehension by the Ministry of Social Services' (Sunny Hill Hospital Tertiary Task Force, 1993, p. 4). The Sunny Hill Tertiary Task Force notes that approximately 60 per cent of the infants admitted to the in-patient program at Sunny Hill Hospital were Native Indian (Sunny Hill Tertiary Task Force, 1993, p. 7), and only one-third of the infants transferred to the NAS in-patient program were returned to their birth parents following discharge (Lauridsen-Hoegh, 1991, p. 13). As one Native mother interviewed noted:

I noticed. I used to read the names every day to see if there was a white baby. There are never really any. And I really looked at it good one day and I noticed, all Native. I said, 'Look, all Native babies.' [Grace]

A follow-up program was also developed through Sunny Hill Hospital to assess these infants developmentally over time, and when parents failed to show for their scheduled appointments the Ministry of Social Services was contacted by hospital staff.

Community representatives (Native Indian and non-Native) pointed out how difficult it was for some parents to understand the hospital process, and that the poverty in the parents' lives often made it difficult for them to travel to the hospital. As well, they pointed out how difficult it was for Native Indian parents who were themselves victimized through government policy, such as residential schools, to interact with social workers and medical professionals (Sunny Hill Tertiary Task Force, 1993).

Historically, women of colour have been denied the right to mother their own children in North America (Collins, 1994; Gupta, 1995; Wong, 1994). Although the ideology of mothering in Western society portrays women as maternal and giving, women of colour are portrayed in more negative terms. They have been perceived by the state as incapable of caring for their own children (Gupta, 1995). Native Indian women have rarely been allowed the right to raise their own children in Canada; residential schools, and later the child welfare system, separated children from their families (Gupta, 1995; Monture, 1989). Although Native Indian people represent less than 4 per cent of the population, 51 per cent of the children-in-care in B.C. as a result of court orders are Native Indian (Report of the Aboriginal Committee, 1992, p. 1). The placement of Native Indian infants in the NAS program at Sunny Hill has created a new avenue for child apprehension by the Ministry of Social Services and the medical profession (see Lauridsen-Hoegh, 1991, p. 13; Sunny Hill Tertiary Task Force, 1993, p. 7).

Although Sunny Hill Hospital recognized that the mothers who have infants at the NAS program were often single parents who have few social supports, resources were allocated in the past to create a therapeutic foster parent support group, rather than a birth parent group; and the NAS program coordinator expressed concern about providing support to grieving foster parents when NAS infants were returned to the birth parents (Lauridsen-Hoegh 1991, p. 16). The grief that birth parents might experience when their infant was transferred to the NAS program and the additional grief they experienced when their infants were placed in temporary or permanent foster care were not acknowledged.

The close liaison between the NAS program at Sunny Hill Hospital and the Ministry of Social Services had other negative effects on families involved in the program. Family court often relied on medical testimony from Sunny Hill in determining custody cases of infants labelled with NAS. The mothers' needs and feelings were often ignored in family court decisions. The ideological assumptions about the superiority of expert knowledge are applicable to all women, for economic problems have now become medical problems (Arnup, 1994; Davin, 1978; Myers, Olson, & Kaltenbach, 1992; Oakley, 1992). With the advent of the public health and maternal health movements, motherhood has become a medicalized domain.

In addition, ideological assumptions about 'good mothers' are shaped by assumptions about race and class. Familial ideology recognizes only white, middle-class, nuclear family arrangements as the norm; all other family forms are typically unrecognized by social workers and family court judges (Chunn & Gavigan, 1991).

The founding director of the Sunny Hill NAS program noted that, when infants were temporarily or permanently apprehended by the Ministry of Social Services, the mother would appear in family court:

Then they would appear in court and I would be called on as an expert witness and ... in the normal pursuit of the justice system, if this was being contested by mum, then she would have some medical expert to present a challenge, but there wasn't anybody you see ... I was sensitive to the fact that this was an uneven playing field for them. I'm the expert, nobody knew how to challenge me in court. I'd be cross examined ... not effectively, and ah ... because they, I knew everything there was to know. And the counsel for the mum would tend to just throw me off, to ask me questions just to have me lose my temper. And I don't have a temper to lose. It's a waste of time. So with that imbalance I'm very careful not to say this baby should or should not go home. I merely describe the baby's special needs. I don't usually know the mum that well to be passing judgment anyway. So I describe the special needs. Then I leave it to the social worker, who knows mum better than I anyway to help the court decide whether that mother is capable of providing for those needs. [1]

Chunn and Menzies (1990) note that judges accept the expertise of medical professionals in court. However, medical professionals hold assumptions about 'morality, sexuality and family life' that reinforce and reproduce patriarchal relations (Chunn & Menzies, 1990, p. 50). Consequently, women who cannot conform to the norm are punished. Because the NAS in-patient program is the only one of its kind in B.C., an opposing opinion was lacking. Judges in family court found it difficult to assess the safety of the children labelled NAS, and medical criteria developed by Sunny Hill Hospital were given more weight than other information (Sunny Hill Tertiary Task Force, 1993). Furthermore, the Sunny Hill Tertiary Task Force report notes that the information gathered from the NAS in-patient program was lacking in context (1993, p. 7). Thus, family court decisions were primarily shaped by the 'expert' opinion of Sunny Hill Hospital, according to criteria they had constructed.

Sunny Hill Hospital staff have has been given the label 'baby snatchers' by many communities in the Lower Mainland, and (as 'Jill' reported) women claim that they are 'petrified' of the medical director of the NAS program. Some of the mothers consented to having their children transferred to Sunny Hill. But when consent was lacking, infants were apprehended by the Ministry of Social Services. One of the mothers interviewed was unaware of the ministry's involvement with Sunny Hill Hospital. She describes her contact with Sunny Hill:

He was born and then put in a special care unit at Children's Hospital. The last couple of days that he was there that's when the director got involved and that was when he basically scared me half to death. So I thought 'Well okay, I better do this then.' He did tell me that once he was sent to Sunny Hill that social services would become involved and I had never had any dealings with social services as far as a social worker. I had been on welfare before and knew I could deal with financial workers. I didn't know the power social workers had over your life. And that was one of the worst mistakes I believe I ever made in my life. I immediately lost total power over what happened to my child, what I needed to do. I just lost total power over everything. Everything from that point on was dictated to me. And it was sort of, I felt a real – with the risk or sounding paranoid – a bit of a conspiracy between the social worker and the director of Sunny Hill. [Greta]

Lack of Alternative Information about NAS Treatment Regimes

The NAS program at Sunny Hill was based on the care of the infants. Outside of telling parents how to bathe and feed their infants, no instructions were offered to parents. If mothers failed to do these jobs properly, the ministry was contacted. The past director of the NAS program states:

We have an opportunity to, if parents come in, to first of all ... teach them how to bathe the baby and feed them. And if they seem to bathe them in a very objectionable way then the social worker would be apprised. [1]

Mothers' mistakes were reported, which contributed to an environment that was often perceived as hostile to the mother. The medicalization of mothering has emphasized surveillance, rather than care (Arnup, 1994; Davin, 1978; Mitchinson, 1988; Oakley, 1986). Mothers who cannot learn to feed and bathe their infants according to the director's instructions are perceived as 'bad mothers' who need to be monitored by the ministry.

Though many of the mothers questioned the care their children received, they were not knowledgeable about other treatment protocols, and had no access to outside information about NAS:

I didn't know ... I questioned the program ... a lot ... at the time, I remember feeling that there was not anything wrong with her. She seemed like a very normal baby to me. Even to the point where I didn't think she really needed all that quiet room and stuff ... I didn't see anything too much wrong with her. It is kind of a sensory deprivation there. That they are doing up there. Which ... see, I have never actually seen really affected drug- babies either. So, I couldn't say that the treatment that they were giving her was right or wrong. Because I had never seen the symptoms. [Pat]

Another mother stated:

We didn't know what anybody ... we didn't know maybe what they were doing in Calgary, or what they were doing in Montreal, or whatever. We didn't know anyone else's research. We only knew what they told us at Sunny Hill and it was taken as God's word, kind of thing, because of course they know and they have got your baby. That's the biggie. [Donna]

Of course, the fact that Sunny Hill did 'have the baby' made all the difference. Another mother described how she personalized her infant's lack of care at Sunny Hill:

I took it on as a personal thing that she wasn't getting cuddled; that she wasn't getting loved ... Because of the format there ... I mean, how could I really expect a bunch of strangers to give something to her that I couldn't give to her myself. So, I probably had a lot of issues involved but I personalized it. It wasn't the doctors or the nurses that weren't providing something for her ... I mean it was my fault that she was there. That is the way that I viewed those things ... I felt responsible for everything that was going on in my life. [Pat]

The majority of the mothers interviewed considered the care of their infants their primary responsibility; in this respect, they adhered to the ideology of mothering that prevails in Western society. So they often personalized any harm, or suspected harm, their infants experienced due to NAS, or their confinement at Sunny Hill. It is not surprising that mothers were often reluctant to challenge the medical staff at Sunny Hill concerning the care of their infants. Most felt guilty about their drug use, and feared that if they raised any objection to the way their infants were cared for they might be perceived as troublemakers and this might jeopardize their chances of having their infants returned to them.

Patient Release and Follow-up

After the infants were released from the in-patient program, they generally spent about two days in the lit children's nursery and then were sent home or to a foster care placement. Specific follow-up instructions were given to mothers and foster caretakers. Instructions were to be followed strictly, and when mothers did not follow them the ministry was contacted by Sunny Hill. For single mothers, and poor women, the follow-up instructions presented many problems.

Prior to the discharge of any infant from the in-patient program, a conference was held. The special needs of the infant were explained to the parent or foster caretaker. The discharge meeting was attended by the Sunny Hill paediatrician, the medical director of the NAS program, the parents or foster caretakers, community health nurse, a ministry social worker, Sunny Hill Hospital social worker, Sunny Hill's NAS clinic nurse-coordinator, and any other health care professionals or support workers involved with the family (Sunny Hill Hospital, 1992b). When there were child protection concerns, or the infant had already been apprehended by the ministry, the ministry was considered the primary stakeholder at the conference. The discharge conference was *not* held if the infant was discharged to an experienced foster caretaker. Rather, a community health nurse informed the foster caretaker and the ministry of the infant's needs.

The Sunny Hill follow-up care guidelines listed the following areas of concern: sudden infant death syndrome (SIDS), poor resistance to infection, medications, screaming, secondary withdrawal, community health nurse follow-up, developmental follow-up, and medical follow-up (Sunny Hill Hospital, 1992b). Sunny Hill Hospital believed that the risk of SIDS for infants labelled NAS was eight to ten times higher than for non-drug infants (Sunny Hill Hospital for Children, 1992b). It was believed that the infant needed to sleep in the same place, with the same time patterns, and the infant needed to be in a smoke-free environment; all cigarette smoking was to take place outside. Immunizations were delayed to six months of age (though this policy was under review in 1992).

The founding director of the NAS program at Sunny Hill describes his medical protocol for protecting NAS infants from sudden infant death syndrome (SIDS):

I'm very strong on keeping the baby at home, developing regular sleep patterns, in the same place. Apparently being in a different bed, a different room, can make enough difference. And whether that has a relationship to SIDS we don't know. But, I'm pretty strong on that and a few other points which are hunches on my part. So far none of them are proven. [1]

In contrast to these views, many researchers claim that there is little or no relationship between maternal illicit drug use and SIDS (Brown & Zuckerman, 1991; Hepburn, 1993a; Humphries, 1993; Mayes et al., 1992).

The founding director at Sunny Hill claimed:

There is animal evidence for a susceptibility to infection, for animals that were born to mothers who were given drugs during their pregnancy. [1]

It was believed that infants labelled NAS had poor resistance to infection; therefore, these infants were not allowed to go to 'shopping malls, churches, health clinics or anywhere there may be unnecessary contacts' (Sunny Hill Hospital for Children, 1992b, p. 2). Contact with other people besides the primary caretaker was limited. The fact that the infants were exposed to many different medical staff during their stay at the in-patient NAS program was not addressed. The nurses who cared for the infants were on shifts. Therefore, infants might have three different nurses caring for them in one day, and these nurses might not work consistent days or nights. Consequently, the next day the infants might be exposed to a new set of nurses. Upon an infant's release from Sunny Hill, the founding director advocated that:

For the first five or six months, first of all the daycare thing is really out, because that's where people exchange all these viruses ... and if mom has to go shopping at the supermarket it is better to have someone come in, particularly from a SIDS standpoint. [1]

Most of the women were told that they could not take their infants out for one year; this was also confirmed by many foster caretakers who had NAS infants. However, for women who lacked social support and access to financial resources, enforced isolation was difficult to maintain.

None of the infants labelled NAS was allowed any medication, including over-the-counter medication, unless it was authorized by a doctor. It was also claimed that these infants labelled NAS might become 'screamers,' developing a high-pitched cry that could last for hours, no matter how much the caregiver attempted to care for them. Mothers and foster parents were instructed that swaddling the infants, protecting them from noise and light, and, most important, having another person available to provide relief for the caretaker would help when the infants became inconsolable (Sunny Hill Hospital, 1992b). These instructions may appear to be helpful; however, most mothers had little access to 'relief,' as a foster parent might.

Sunny Hill Hospital also expressed concern about secondary withdrawal in its follow-up instructions. It was believed that infants labelled NAS might experience a second withdrawal up to six months of age. However this withdrawal might be difficult to detect, for it might 'mimic symptoms of potentially life-threatening diseases' (Sunny Hill Hospital for Children, 1992b, p. 3). Caretakers were advised to go immediately to emergency or contact their family doctor. The founding NAS director claimed:

The secondary withdrawal may be worse than the first, or more often less inten-
sive. And it may take the form of diarrhoea, crankiness, increase in crying at
night, a lot of them, there's a lot of tremors. [1]

When asked how he distinguished between secondary withdrawal and flu,
colic, or normal tremors (as some of the infants are premature), he
responded:

A lot of them are [premature]. Basically, I don't think we bat a hundred in differ-
entiating here. If the baby's showing signs, then the chances are the signs will dis-
appear if we went in for the darkened room for a few nights and that kind of
thing. In other words, remove as much of the stimulus as possible. [1]

This response does not establish whether secondary withdrawal actually
exists. The symptoms described are exhibited in healthy children who
have not been exposed to maternal drug use (Morrison & Siney, 1996;
Weston, Ivins, Zuckerman, Jones, & Lopez, 1989). As well, most infant illnesses will subside within a few days. So is it the passage of time or the
darkened room and the administration of opiates that is effective? Is it a
normal infant illness or secondary withdrawal that the baby experiences?
The fact that the symptoms subside while the infant is in the darkened
room does not establish the fact of secondary withdrawal.

Mothers were given all of the instructions noted above prior to discharge of their babies. The 'special needs' of these 'at risk' infants were
often both frightening and difficult to care for. The whole structure of
the mothers' lives changed when their infants were released to go
home:

They told us we had to really be careful with him, not to have loud noises like TV,
music ... what else was there? And we had to keep him like in a dim, dark room.
Not as dark as the one in the hospital, though. [Lori]

They gave you these rules and regulations when you bring him home. How to
care for him, how to approach him, how to touch him, how to keep him wrapped
tight. To avoid the noise, the TV and vacuum cleaner and stuff like that. Loud
groups of people and stuff like that. I was just scared. Everything the paper told
me to do for NAS, it was like I can't just go out, I can't take my son out, I can't go
visit my family ... I was just so afraid because I couldn't go anywhere, I had no
transportation. I couldn't take my baby on the bus, couldn't do anything. Take
him to the store. I mean, it was like I was locked in this place, and the place I had

was just half of this whole space, one little bedroom, one little living room with a kitchen. [Ellie]

For the mothers interviewed, the follow-up guidelines were very difficult to adhere to. Their lives became very regimented and isolated, and the support that they might have received from friends and family members was no longer an option, given the rigid medical rules surrounding contact, crowds, and visiting.

Much of the care and medical protocol established by the founding director at the NAS program at Sunny Hill was based on 'hunches,' based in turn on ideological assumptions, rather than scientific evidence. Nevertheless, the mothers had to comply with the established medical protocol, for fear of losing their children to the ministry. As the founding director observed:

The fear of my helping the court to have them lose their baby, that's a real threat ... More and more mothers have learned not to get into the net [to come to the attention of medical professions] because of the fear of their baby being apprehended. [1]

Although the mothers' fear of apprehension by the ministry was recognized, it was not addressed within the NAS program at Sunny Hill. Rather, child apprehensions were considered to be justified, due to the infants' special needs, and the program was not modified to welcome mothers rather than frightening them away.

Follow-up Assessment

All of the infants were given their first developmental assessment at four months of age and the last one at eight years of age. These assessments were conducted at Sunny Hill Hospital by 'specialized therapists,' and the infants were assessed at the NAS Medical Follow-up Clinic at Sunny Hill (Sunny Hill Hospital, 1992b). Follow-up appointments were often stressful for both mothers and children. One Native Indian mother stated:

The first check-up with me, we were in the treatment centre. And it was really, it was really stressful for me and for them ... I didn't know what was gonna happen; they didn't tell me what was gonna happen. We all just went into these rooms, and they separated the boys. And the people who drove me to Sunny Hill, they had to stay with J. in one room, and we were in the other room, me and G. And so J. was getting real scared because he didn't know anybody. And it was just the people who drove us there, and it was real scary for him so he wasn't participating with them ... sixteen months [old], he didn't know anyone. So they left the door open, and they were both in the same room, and they were both screaming ... And it was really hard, and all my stress went to the small of my back. And oh, I felt real small because of what they were asking me, 'cause I don't know how to play with my kids or nothing. [Jill]

[They are] sixteen months. I don't know where they get off saying that they are the way of a thirteen-month-old. Just because, I heard this one guy on the bus when the babies were babies right, they were small, he said they didn't start walking till they were seventeen months old, his child. And thirteen, fourteen months my boys were walking, and it made me happy because the guy said his baby didn't start walking until he was seventeen months old. And so every baby is different. I don't know where they get off in trying to test them, like they are testing. If they test another baby whose mother never used drugs or alcohol or smoked, [it] probably would be worse than what these guys were. [Jill]

After release from the NAS in-patient program, the mothers and infants were visited by community health nurses in their homes until the infants were eleven months old. The nurses were instructed to measure the infants' weight, length, and head circumference, and to monitor for SIDS and silent otitis media (inflammation of the middle ear), which they believed occurred more often in infants labelled with NAS. Any deviation from the usual growth curve was considered a possible sign of 'impending SIDS' (Lauridsen-Hoegh, 1991, p. 16). The founding director claimed that the public health nurses

picked up things we wouldn't here, seeing the baby in the home ... and the nurses were terrific, they would phone me if there was nobody home when they got there or if they were having problems. [1]

The surveillance of the mother's behaviour continued long after her infant was released from the program.

The community health nurse provided duplicate copies of the NAS flow sheet to the family doctor of the parents or foster caretakers, at her own discretion (Sunny Hill Hospital, 1992b). For all the medical concern expressed for these infants, parents were not offered any type of parenting or support group to educate them or to lend them support, either when their infants were in the in-patient program or later when they came home. For some parents, the infants never did come home, but were placed in foster care. Lauridsen-Hoegh claims that only one-third of the infants went home to their parents, and many of these children would spend a period of time in foster care first. The rest of the infants were 'adopted as special-needs children' (1991, p. 15).

The fear of infants being apprehended by the ministry was present at all times. Although an infant might be able to return to the birth parents' home upon discharge, mothers were not secure that this arrangement would continue. Community health nurses and Sunny Hill Hospital contacted the ministry whenever a mother failed to show up for an appointment, or when they had child-protection concerns. As one mother stated:

There would be nothing I could be caught at. But I was still really paranoid, so I was over cautious about following by their rules ... Not to go to crowded places, no noises, keeping her structured. [Donna]

Although mothers attempted to follow the instructions laid out by Sunny Hill Hospital, there was no guarantee that this would be enough to ensure that their children would not be apprehended after discharge. One mother expressed her frustration about the community health nurse's visit. Her child always became upset when the nurse undressed, weighed, and measured him. The mother began to undress the child herself during the visits because he was more tolerant of her touch. One day she left her infant in her mother's care during a community health nurse visit. She describes the visit:

So one day she came to do her whole trip and my mom was there. So my son was really agitated when she went to do her procedure. And she went and reported to the director that J. seemed really agitated today and I wasn't there. The director wrote a letter to my social worker and said to her that if anything ... my son was high-risk and if he died my son's blood would be on her hands. They thought the baby was going to die. That was a crock, Susan, it really was. I really watched my son, and really got to know my son. I was with him as much as I could be with him during that time. Out of guilt I wanted to see how much damage I could detect, so I really got to know my baby, you know, and it wasn't true. He was really a fairly normal baby except for the diarrhoea ... as soon as he [the director] got that note from the health nurse, he just turned on me like I couldn't believe. [Greta]

The medical staff at Sunny Hill, the community health nurse, and social services accepted that the infant's care always took precedence over the mother's concerns.

Resistance

All of the mothers interviewed whose children were sent to Sunny Hill Hospital were on social assistance, with little access to other economic and social supports. Unequal power relations between the mothers and the medical and social service professionals, the mothers' economic situation, isolation, and a lack of formal education, often contributed to difficulties in negotiating with the medical and social work professionals involved in their infants' lives. Often what appeared to be a minor incident to the staff at Sunny Hill would be quite traumatic to the mother involved. One mother describes an incident at Sunny Hill when her son was there:

I was coming down with the flu. I had a headache; I could feel the cold coming on and I thought if I take two aspirins then I'd be okay. But when I got to the nurses' station and asked, 'Can I get two Tylenols, or two aspirin?' and they said no. And I said, 'What do you mean no, this is a hospital. I know you have Tylenol in there.' And they said, 'No, you can't have it.' I said, 'I can't believe this. I have one more feeding before I can go home, and ... I don't want to have to go all the way to Burnaby.' And they said, 'We can't give it to you.' So I called my mom, and said, 'Mom, can I come and get two aspirins?' She said sure.
   So I had to go home. And I made explicit arrangements with the nurse that I would be back in two hours to feed my son, and not to feed him till I got there. They said, 'Yeah, okay, no problem.' So I went to my mom's, and came back. And in between I missed the bus ... I kept calling the hospital and saying 'I'm coming, so don't feed my son.' And when I got there, she was feeding my son. Well, I just went into a rage. 'I thought I told you not to feed my son.' So we got into an argument. So I stomped out of there, looking for the social worker, or whoever, to say, 'Why did you do this?'
   And [the social worker] was at a conference in Chicago, and they got her on the phone: 'We've got this raging woman and we want her out of here.' And they had the maintenance man and the security standing there in front of the door and the women standing there holding my baby. [Telling me] 'You get out of here, you don't belong here.' I was so upset, I said, 'Lady, you have my baby in your hands; you put my baby down now.' And she was screaming at me, and I was screaming back at her. And I went to walk back in and the security said, 'Please come out; you are disturbing the other babies.' And I said, 'Right,' and I walked

out. She was still standing there with my baby in her hands, saying 'You get out of here.' And I said, 'Lady, you better put my baby down.' And finally she put my baby down. And I said, 'Don't ever talk to me that way with my baby in your arms.' And I told her, 'I have the right to be here anytime I want to be.'

I was just furious. I think I still have what I said and what she said on a piece of paper, because I knew that this wasn't right. [Ellie]

Many of the mothers discussed the positive support they received from one of the social workers at Sunny Hill. Unfortunately, this social worker was not always available, and could not change medical protocol. Nevertheless, her support was invaluable to many mothers who had few advocates and limited options.

Although the mothers interviewed were often powerless to directly challenge the medical care of their infants at Sunny Hill, they were not passive. Rogers and Buffalo (1974) note how people develop techniques to fight against bureaucracies. Similarly, the women interviewed individually resisted interference in caring for their infants as much as possible, given the relatively powerless situation they were in (i.e., that if a mother did not comply with the experts, her child was usually apprehended by the ministry). One mother describes her initial visit with the founding director of Sunny Hill immediately after she gave birth to her son at Grace Hospital:

He came in with a little beard, whiskers showing, and no teeth and I had my son with me and I was in the room by myself. It was dark, nine o'clock. The baby was sleeping, and I was there, and I was just happy. And then he came in and just freaked me out. No white jacket or anything to identify him. And I said, 'Who are you?' And he said, 'The director.' And at that point I didn't remember ... the name of the doctor that was going to come see me. So I said to him, 'Can I see your driver's licence?' So he showed me his driver's licence, but that still didn't mean that he was a doctor. He said, 'I understand, it's quite all right.' So when he walked out I followed him, and I saw through the window that he was behind where the counter is and he was talking to the nurse. And I thought 'Oh my god! This doctor is so busy, and I threw him out!' [Ellie]

Often mothers chose to resist specific instructions they did not agree with and attempted to create loving relationships with their infants despite the institutional setting at Sunny Hill. Several mothers described their attempts to care for their infants there:

And there was no talking to them ... We were not supposed to, but we did ... They told us to just keep it quiet in there. I know a lot of times I wanted to laugh when I was in there, because you know, I put a big diaper on C., and it came under her armpits. I couldn't help but to laugh. We used to visit one little girl that was a mixture of white and Chinese in there too, so every time the nurse was gone and she cried, we would visit with her too and give her [a] soother ... they were the two noisiest ones in there after a while. They would talk to each other and you could hear them laugh. I guess we kind of stimulated both of them. You know, built them up. [Grace]

The whole thing was that they made you feel really scared to touch your baby. But I loved my baby, and I'm going to touch him and I'm going to be there. [Ellie]

No, they let me hold her and part of that was because I was aware that she was borderline after talking to [the director]. They tried that on me a few times, the quiet room and no this and no that ... 'Leave the baby. Don't get the baby agitated.' Well ... my argument, I think it is pretty agitating for the baby not to be held. It is really agitating for me not to be held, so I am getting held. [Pat]

The mothers attempted to incorporate their own values and parenting skills whenever possible, regardless of the rules and medical protocol they were told to follow both at Sunny Hill and at home. As described above, the mothers touched and spoke to their babies when nurses were out of the room, and when they were allowed to bring their infants home some of them disregarded the follow-up rules. Their resistance to medical protocol was not due to ignorance or passive aggression; it was an acknowledgment of their own beliefs, values, parenting skills, and assessments of their infants' needs, which often differed from those of the staff at Sunny Hill, community health nurses, and social workers. Although the mothers lacked medical training, their assessments of their children's needs appeared to be fairly accurate, and reasonable.

It's the Drugs!

Other mothers whose infants had not been labelled with NAS, but who had a history of drug use, expressed concern that, due to their past history of drug use, doctors failed to search for other reasons for their infants' ailments. Morrison and Siney (1996) also discovered that symptoms exhibited by infants being monitored for NAS are automatically attributed to withdrawal. One mother's infant was quite jittery a few weeks after birth. Her doctor assumed her infant was experiencing withdrawal and suggested giving the infant tranquillizers. She stated:

It just didn't seem right with me and I ended up going ... in the Fairmont building. This big red-haired doctor ... he suggested taking him off milk and putting him on soya bean milk. Well, it was like day and night ... Because he was a drug baby I don't think the other doctor ... they don't look to other things. [Linda]

Another mother discussed her concern when she visited her doctor on three separate occasions because her child appeared to be having difficulty breathing:

I undressed her, because I assumed she was going to be, you know, examined. And he didn't. He just sat at his desk and he says, 'Oh now, it is just the methadone. It will pass.' It was then that I got another doctor ... I explained what was happening, and that was at 12:30 at night. And he says, 'Meet me, at the Children's Hospital ... now' ... and she had pneumonia in her left lung. [Evelyn]

Other mothers whose children had not been diagnosed at birth with NAS were now being told that their children's later illnesses might be due to maternal drug use. One Native mother states:

It was suggested [by nurses at Children's Hospital] that my daughter's asthma could be from my drug abuse. I don't know, that could be inherited, or brought on by stress. [Cathy]

It was also suggested by the nurses at Children's Hospital that this same mother's four-year-old twins might have NAS:

Signs are just coming out right now with their behaviour problems and hyperactivity [Cathy].

Mothers reported being advised by daycare workers, teachers, social workers, nurses, and doctors that behavioural and physiological symptoms that their children displayed were signs of NAS. These professionals did not consider the effects of economic and social deprivation. Maternal drug use and the failure of the mothers to protect their children were perceived as the root of the children's problems. Rather than search for more complex answers, the social and health care professionals involved in the lives of mothers and children labelled NAS act according to ideologies that misrepresent maternal drug use, mothering, and poverty.

Conclusion

Although mothers often individually disagreed with the medical protocols developed at the NAS program at Sunny Hill Hospital, no significant changes occurred. The new director of the NAS program at Sunny Hill has established new policy, although it is too soon to evaluate the changes in the program.

In the past, mothers who challenged rules and policy were often perceived as non-compliant by the staff at Sunny Hill. Child apprehensions by the ministry were seen as justifiable due to the infants' special needs and at-risk status. However, NAS special needs and medical criteria were developed by Sunny Hill Hospital, and there were no other medical professionals available to challenge them in family court. So mothers were at increased risk of child apprehension by the ministry once their infants were transferred to the NAS program at Sunny Hill. Despite the fact that many infants transferred there were not exhibiting signs of NAS but rather had been transferred for other reasons, including a lack of foster care placement.

Furthermore, medical treatment in the care of the infants labelled with NAS was often based on experimental treatment and 'hunches' lacking in scientific validity. These 'hunches' were based on ideological assumptions concerning mothering, illicit drug use, and poverty. Many of the mothers believed that the long periods of isolation, darkness, and sensory deprivation to which their children were subjected were a form of punishment and child abuse, rather than medical treatment. Medical personnel at Sunny Hill often contacted the Ministry of Social Services about mothers' perceived non-compliance. The mothers rarely had advocates to whom they could turn to with their own concerns.

Overall, the medical treatment of NAS infants at Sunny Hill, the darkened rooms, the sensory deprivation, the length of stay, the forced feeding, the lack of contact with families, the failure to provide mothers with a clear and understandable protocol to follow, the fear of child apprehension, the surveillance and control of mothers, and the ideology of the founding director of the NAS program contributed to an environment of hostility towards the mothers and experimental treatment of their infants. It would be difficult to distinguish long-term developmental problems due to maternal drug use from the effects of infants' length of residence in such an environment. At the least, these infants were denied contact with their families, and the mothers deprived of their infants. How much damage was done to these infants during their stay has never been established.

What is most telling is that the ten infants in this study transferred to the NAS program came from families on social assistance, that 40 per cent were Native Indian and 70 per cent of the children were eventually permanently apprehended by the Ministry of Social Services. The practice of inflicting inherently punitive and experimental medical treatment on vulnerable communities has an extensive history in North America. Since 1992 the program at Sunny Hill has been revised. The Sunny Hill Tertiary Task Force (1993) was critical of the NAS program, and the new director has made changes. This suggests that the mothers were not alone in their assessment of the NAS program at Sunny Hill.

Medical models of care that use their own criteria to establish 'risk' and 'special needs' have increased the social control and surveillance of mothers by monitoring the care of their infants. Once an infant has been taken away for in-patient medical treatment, his or her mother has few options outside of complying with treatment protocols if she wishes to have her infant returned to her. Mothers are monitored and controlled, and if they do not comply with medical advice they are punished.

Historically, poor women and women of colour have often been denied the chance to mother their own children. In the treatment of NAS at Sunny Hill Hospital, mothers were denied the chance to care for their own children. The promise of the return of their children was used as an enticement to enforce compliance with a medical program embedded in class, gender, and race biases. This program failed to address the real needs and social context of both infant and mother. Programs that exclusively subscribe to medical models of care, as opposed to client-centred and client-directed programs, disregard the social realm in invoking science to justify their policies.

4

Social Services: Intervention and Regulation

Women are vulnerable to social service intervention, even when their children have not been labelled NAS. Women in Canada who use illicit drugs are often challenged by social services agencies in relation to their mothering. Single mothers who use illicit drugs are much more likely to come into contact with social services than are men (Cain, 1994). Many social service professionals equate illicit drug use with poor mothering (Humphries et al., 1992; Maher, 1992; Maier, 1992), which places children at risk at birth or later in life. In addition, social work agencies have expanded their control to define and act in specific cases where foetal harm is suspected (Gómez, 1994). The apprehension of children of any age, and the reduction or denial of services, are interventions used by social workers to regulate women's behaviour.

Contemporary Social Services

Today social welfare legislation arises out of a 'politically conservative anti-drug ideology' that emulates legal and medical interests (Kasinsky, 1994, p. 121), especially in the United States. Historically, and in the current North American context, the interests of the mother and child 'have been perceived by the state as separate, and often in conflict with each other' (Kasinsky, 1994, p. 98).

Social workers' power lies in their ability to label women 'deviant' (Amir & Biniamin, 1992), and 'deserving and undeserving' (Chunn, 1995). The assessment of mothering and proper female roles is integral to welfare policy (Edwards, 1988; Maher, 1992; Maier, 1992). Currently, women who receive welfare are often portrayed as an underclass of uneducated, single parents who are out of control, unfit, sexually promiscuous, cunning, who have children to continue to receive welfare benefits, and who regularly cheat the welfare system (Gorlick, 1995; Martin, 1991). These misapplied characteristics dominate conservative discourse concerning women and welfare benefits.

In contrast, Gorlick's (1995) study of single parents emphasizes the diversity of women on welfare assistance in Canada. Seeing women as unfit, helpless, and overwhelmed deflects attention away from the 'feminization of poverty,' an increase in families headed by women which may be attributed to their role of providing most of the support for their children, and their disadvantage in the labour market (Pearce, 1990, p. 267).

Assistance that barely (or rarely) covers the basic necessities, and the stigma of welfare, make assistance less than appealing for most women. But, most important, receiving assistance opens the door to surveillance by social service agencies. Women are judged according to their fitness to care for their families and their adherence to feminine virtue.

Foster caretakers receive up to three times as much financial assistance from the B.C. Ministry of Social Services for each child they care for as mothers on financial aid receive. They are also offered additional services, such as counselling for the children and respite care. Mothers are rarely offered such services. Traditionally, mothers are refused additional support by the ministry, whether in terms of a homemaker, daycare (unless they are attending school full-time), or counselling, unless there is an open file and a social worker has been assigned to the case (Report of the Aboriginal Committee, 1992, p. 46). Having an open file and social worker, rather than just a financial worker, means that the woman is subjected to a 'child protection' concern by the social worker (The People's Law School, 1993). In short, mothers are not offered assistance until their families are in a state of crisis, and preventive support is rarely offered prior to family breakdown.

In Canada, when social workers think that a child is unsafe or neglected, they can have the child removed, which is called 'child apprehension' (Ministry of Social Services, 1996). Social workers do not need proof that a child is 'in need of protection'; they can act on their own assumptions (Report of the Aboriginal Committee, 1992, p. 67). The rights of the child and the power of the ministry supersede the rights of the parents (The People's Law School, 1993). Canadian society includes many different cultures with many different ideas about the best way to care for children. But social workers have little or no training in cultural awareness. When they are sent out to observe behaviour and to assess a situation in a home, they bring all their ethnocentric cultural baggage with them (Almonte, 1994). This is not to say that children are not in need of protection – they are. It has been demonstrated that some families are unable to care for their children and seek assistance from the ministry (Ministry of Social Services, 1992, p. 22). As well, incidents of child abuse have been reported and substantiated (Ministry of Social Services, 1992, p. 21).

Traditionally, social workers have been white, middle-class women, though there are male social workers too, especially in administrative positions. Making decisions about people's families, especially across cultures, can be fraught with difficulties. The social worker may not be aware of what certain behaviours mean in that culture (Almonte, 1994). An action that the parents perceive as part of fulfilling their parental roles may be interpreted as abuse.

Child Apprehension

Child apprehension, whether temporary or permanent, is one tool that the welfare system wields when a mother is deemed unfit or undeserving. In Canada, child-welfare laws define and legislate what is considered 'good parenting' (Pulkingham, 1994, p. 92). Social workers and the courts, through child-welfare law, 'intrude into the so-called "private sphere" of many families' (Pulkingham, 1994, p. 92). And it is poor women and women of colour, and especially First Nations women, who are most likely to be scrutinized and to have their children apprehended by the Ministry of Social Services and sent to foster care.

An emerging body of critical research sceptical of the foster care system has developed (see Gupta, 1995; Hawley & Disney, 1992; Humphries et al., 1992; Maher, 1992; Noble, 1997; Report of the Aboriginal Committee, 1992; Chavkin, Allen, & Oberman, 1991; Monture, 1989). These authors highlight the surveillance and intervention of social services in the lives of poor women and women of colour in Western societies.

First Nations Children

Most child and foetal apprehension in the United States occurs with First Nations, Latinas, and black women (Maier, 1992). In Canada, of the children in care, First Nations children are overrepresented (Report of the Aboriginal Committee, 1992; Monture, 1989). Although First Nations people represent less than 4 per cent of the population, 51 per cent of the children in care as a result of court orders under the Family and

Child Service Act in British Columbia are First Nations, and 13.5 per cent of children voluntarily in care are First Nations children (Report of the Aboriginal Committee, 1992, p. 1). Alberta, Saskatchewan, and Manitoba have even higher rates of First Nations children in care (Monture, 1989). Over a generation, more than one out of five First Nations children has become a ward of the court in British Columbia (Report of the Aboriginal Committee, 1992, p. 2). Faith also notes that 'many younger Native women in Canada's jails and prisons have been raised in foster or adoptive homes which, in effect, have been an extension of the residential school policies' (1993, p. 198).

The Report of the Aboriginal Committee (1992) states that children were apprehended because Native culture did not fit white, middle-class values and norms. Social workers had no understanding of the complexity of the concepts family and extended family within First Nations communities (Report of the Aboriginal Committee, 1992). The lack of running water was sufficient reason to apprehend a child. It was interpreted as being in the 'best interests of the child' to take Native children away from their families and communities and place them in non-aboriginal families, where dominant cultural values could be learned. This not only disrupted traditional Native family structure, but also fostered a 'new industry: the fostering of Aboriginal children' (Report of the Aboriginal Committee, 1992, p. 19). The scope of the child apprehensions that occurred within the Native community is illustrated in the Report of the Aboriginal Committee, which notes that in 1955 in British Columbia, only 1 per cent of children in care were Native, whereas by 1960, 40 per cent were native (1992, p. 20).

Foetal Rights and Social Services

In Canada, the social service industry has extended its interest from live children to the developing foetus. Several legal case studies emphasize the growing concern about foetal rights among the medical and social service professions. In both *Re 'Children's Aid Society for the District of Kenora and J.L.'* (1981) and *Re 'Children's Aid Society of City of Belleville and T et al'* (1987), the courts concluded that the unborn foetuses apprehended were 'children' in need of protection. In *Re 'Baby R'* (1988) a pregnant woman's foetus was apprehended. The mother was pressured into giving consent to a caesarean moments before the surgery was to begin. What is relevant is that the child that was apprehended was not yet born. These were precedent-setting cases in Canada at the time, for the term 'child' under the Family and Child Service Act was open to debate and redefinition. However, under appeal, the court upheld that 'child' referred to children that have been delivered in the *Re 'Baby R'* (1988) case. The foetus can therefore not become a ward of the court. The above apprehensions occurred when mothers failed to comply with medical advice or when social services believed the mother to be unfit to care for the unborn child.

Recently, the Supreme Court of Canada agreed to hear an appeal brought by the Winnipeg's Child and Family Services agency which wanted to force a woman into drug treatment to protect her unborn foetus. The Winnipeg Child and Family Services believed that she was harming her unborn child due to solvent use. This case was perceived as a test case concerning foetal and maternal rights (Roberts, 1996, p. A2). In contrast to U.S. policy, on 31 October 1997, the Supreme Court of Canada ruled that the courts cannot order the detention and treatment of pregnant women to protect the unborn child and that the unborn child does not possess legal rights (Winnipeg Child and Family Services [*Northwest Area v. G. (D.F.)*, 1997]).

Feminists have noted emerging Canadian and U.S child welfare legislation which attempts to define the foetus as a 'child in need of protection' (Chavkin, 1992; Fitzgerald, 1993; Maher, 1992; Maier, 1992; Noble, 1997). These attempts are precedent-setting in their implications for all women, and especially women who use illegal drugs.

The Medicalization of Maternal Drug Use

The interrelationship between the medical and legal professions both informs welfare policy and extends its jurisdiction (Gómez, 1994; Noble, 1997). The power that social service agencies have over women and children is explored by Maher (1992) in relation to women who are suspected of using drugs. Maher (1992) examines how welfare policy enforces dominant norms of womanhood and mothering. She contends that the punishment of women in the United States who use illegal drugs during pregnancy, through arrests and child apprehensions, deflects 'attention away from the fissures of gender, race and class that render these women's lives as publicly problematic' (Maher, 1992, p. 152). She cites urine sampling, treatment centres, apprehensions, fostering, reduced welfare payment, hospital experience, and racial and class discrimination are discussed, as examples of controls employed outside of the legal justice system (Maher, 1992). She concludes that theories of state intervention and legal discourse fail to recognize the way women are controlled through administrative and welfare policy.

Canadian women who use illicit drugs, especially during pregnancy, are also subject to social control. In contrast to the United States, there is no specific social welfare legislation that equates maternal drug use with neglect, or child abuse (Ministry of Social Services, 1996). However, in practice children have been apprehended by the ministry due to their mother's illicit drug use (Sunny Hill Hospital Tertiary Task Force, 1993).

It is well documented that women who use drugs do not seek medical services while pregnant because of their fear of social service intervention and child apprehension (Siney, 1994, 1995; Klee & Lewis, 1994; Hepburn, 1993b). A woman who uses illicit drugs is 'held in contempt by her family, Child Protective Services staff, health professionals and society at large' (Tittle & St. Claire, 1989, p. 18). Of the women interviewed in their three-year study of narcotic users in British Columbia, Stevenson, Lingley, Trasov, & Stansfield (1956) noted that most had children in the care of relatives or social agencies.

In a Vancouver study conducted at Vancouver Children's Hospital between 1952 and 1973, social services were contacted for follow-up information pertaining to 149 children born to 101 women who had used heroin during their pregnancies. Mothers were on welfare during 122 of the deliveries. Over 25 per cent of the women were First Nations women, though Native Indians represented only about 5 per cent of the provincial population at that time (Fricker & Segal, 1978, p. 360). Information was included about an additional 140 children born to the 101 mothers in the study, resulting in a total of 289 children. Only 25 per cent of these children were still living with their mothers; 15.2 per cent were living with relatives and 49.4 were adopted or in foster care (Fricker & Segal, 1978, p. 363).

Foster Care and NAS

The fostering of infants who may have been exposed prenatally to illicit drugs is big business in Canada and the United States. The foster care system is overwhelmed in urban centres. Since 1985, children who have been apprehended in the United States are literally warehoused and given substandard care. In New York City, infants have been kept in hospital wards for months and placed in temporary shelters (Rempel, 1989), such as old school buildings.

In Canada, infants are apprehended after birth if there is suspected maternal drug use, including alcohol use. Although Canada has not progressed to warehousing infants, the foster care system is integral to the lives of Canadian mothers whose children have been labelled with neonatal abstinence syndrome (NAS). Until 1992, medical and welfare services in Vancouver did not offer support groups for mothers whose children were labelled with NAS or FAS (foetal alcohol syndrome). However, Sunny Hill Hospital for Children offered a support group for foster parents who cared for children labelled NAS. Journal articles have devoted space to the trials of the foster parents and those of medical and social service professionals, with little regard for the biological mothers of these infants.

Like other journal articles describing NAS, most articles pertaining to fostering begin with several paragraphs describing the horrors these infants experience after birth. In one of the milder accounts the reader is asked to

imagine a tiny baby whose high-pitched, intense screaming, induced by withdrawal from whatever variety of legal and illegal substances his mother used during pregnancy, goes on hour after hour. Imagine yourself, sitting in a darkened room, trying to feed this underweight newborn, who cannot coordinate sucking, swallowing, and breathing and who therefore gags and chokes after every few sips of fluid. The baby cannot tolerate the stimulus overload of having your arms hold him as he tries desperately to eat. He screams in frustration and fury. Every bit of what he swallowed ends up in your lap. (White, 1992, p. 13)

Evidence negates this kind of description by foster care parents and medical professionals who work with children labelled NAS (see Frank & Zuckerman, 1993; Hepburn, 1993a, 1993b; Latchem, 1994; Morrison & Siney, 1996; Myers et al., 1992; Siney, 1994, 1995; Siney, Kidd, Walkinshaw, Morrison, & Manasse, 1995). These subjective characteristics may fit any infant. Treatment regimens for infants labelled NAS vary. A review of the literature on maternal drug use makes it exceedingly clear that much of the 'care' provided for these infants in North America is experimental.

The apprehension of infants born to mothers suspected of maternal drug use is prevalent in both Canada and the United States (Streissguth, Grant, Ernst, & Phipps, 1994). The medical diagnosis of neonatal abstinence syndrome (NAS) often has a 'cascade effect,' wherein the family is subject to ministry intervention and eventual apprehension of infants. Family court decisions concerning custody of infants also influence criminal court decisions.

Past Social Service History

Seventy-one per cent of the mothers interviewed for this study were receiving social assistance. Of these, 18 per cent were either attending university or college full-time or participating in full-time volunteer work. Social service intervention and ministry apprehension of children can play as much of a role as the criminal law in regulating *poor* women. For poor women and women of colour, social services intersect with medical and criminal justice controls (Gómez, 1994; Humphries et al., 1992; Paltrow, 1992). Maher discusses how welfare policy 'functions as an independent and gender-specific form of punishment and regulation' of women (1992, p. 158). In contrast to the middle-class and professional women in this study who were non-visible illicit drug users, the poor women who were identified as illicit drug users were challenged by social services in relation to their mothering.

In Canada, many social service professionals equate illicit drug use with poor mothering that places children at risk (Cain, 1994). Therefore, many poor women and women of colour, as well as the women in this study, have had their children apprehended by the ministry at birth or later, and placed in temporary or permanent foster care. For those women who were themselves raised in foster care, 'social services' represents oppression. First Nations women define the Canadian welfare system as an extension of the criminal justice system, for both punish people by removing them from their families and communities (Monture, 1989). Social services are also perceived as an extension of the policies reinforced by government residential schools in the past. Many First Nations children were removed from their families and communities and placed in these schools. Foster care in Canada has offered little protection for children. Many children have been moved from one foster home to another. Many have been physically and sexually abused in their foster homes (Report of the Aboriginal Committee, 1992).

Social services intervention in relation to mothers comes in many forms: child apprehension, provision or denial of assistance, crisis grants, surveillance, and forced participation in programs (for example, drug treatment, parenting, and life skills programs). Many of the women interviewed for this study had negative experiences with social services, having been wards of the court in their youth. Some had run away from abusive home situations. Two women of European heritage noted:

I was with my mom, but I ran away. I started running away when I was thirteen. [Julie]

I was so unhappy as a kid, I kept on leaving home. Maybe I should rephrase that. My home was just an empty shell. There was nothing there to hold me. Shooting junk at fourteen gave me a lot more comfort than my home did. Leaving home at fifteen was the best thing I ever did for myself. [Hope]

Rather than turn to social services or other professionals, these women left their home environments. Other women were taken from their families and placed in the care of the ministry. These women discussed the fears related to their own histories as wards of the court, and their fears for their children. One Native Indian mother explained:

You know it was so hard to bond with anybody because we were switched around, home to home ... When that happens like so many times, and finally you do get to a place that you know that you're supposed to settle down at, it's really hard. Because your emotions have been played with, and you're just a kid, right, and you don't know any different. And it's really hard on you. And I think what the ministry's plan was that we'd all be together. And then slowly, one by one, they took us separately away. Yeah. And the youngest ones were adopted out first because younger kids are easier to adopt. I was too old to be adopted, you know ... I always thought that it was the foster parents that were, you know taking me away from my mother ... and I didn't really realize it was the social worker and stuff. I ah, I used to hate when they used to come and take me away. I used to cry all the time. Cry for my mum. I cried for my mum for years and years and years. Used to cry every night. [Sue]

And a woman of European heritage explained:

Yeah, yeah. So, they ended up in social services. Which is a lousy way to grow up. I grew up in Children's Aid. It did me no good. It probably made problems worse for years afterwards. I found no comfort from any home that I ever lived in. No safety, no real life. And I would never want that to happen to my children. You know, I would do anything to avoid that. [Pat]

Some of the women spoke about the physical and sexual abuse they survived while in the care of ministry. Foster parents were not always what they presented to social services. One young woman from a middle-class background who was placed in foster care stated:

And most of these foster homes, they sure put on a good show for social workers and government, but as soon as the worker's out the door and you're left alone, it's like 'You're living in the doghouse and we're keeping up this bedroom for appearances and we make two thousand dollars to have you here.' [Karen]

Two Native Indian women noted:

I really enjoyed it there and I was there for six years, except the only thing that was wrong with it was that I was being abused by them. Physically abused. [Sue]

I was sexually abused ... in a group home. They [social services] ... asked me what I wanted. I said, 'I wanted my real family.' They said, 'Okay, okay, just say in the statement that when you ran away that you made up the statement about the foster father touching you and doing all this other shit to you and breaking your arm. So you write it all up and we'll make sure you get what you want.' And all I wanted was to get out of there. So that's what they did. [Cathy]

Many of the women attempted to resist the abuse they received while in foster care, though their youth and powerless status left few avenues open. One Native Indian woman described her attempt to survive while in foster care:

You know we were disciplined by ... getting the belt, getting punched out, or whatever. That was our discipline. And um, she quit doing it after a while and it was you know the foster dad that was doing it. Finally, you know, I stood up for myself one time and I pulled a knife on him and said, 'Don't come near me, you know I'm tired of this. I've been abused all my life and I'll call the cops on you. You know, I'll call the social worker on you.' So from that day, I never really got ... I did get hit and stuff but ah, not a lot. [Sue]

Aside from physical and sexual abuse, children in the care of the ministry were vulnerable to racism in the foster homes in which they were placed. Monture notes that racism is a form of violence. As a Mohawk woman, she finds racism more difficult to talk about or deal with than sexual and physical violence (Monture-Okanee, Thornhill, & Williams, 1993). She states that 'you can't touch racism, you can't see it, so it's never "real"' (Monture-Okanee et al., 1993). The racism that many of the Native Indian mothers interviewed experienced after they were taken from their homes and communities is evident in their responses:

I grew up in a town where there was a lot of racism. I was adopted by white people who hated Indians. We were more like slaves than kids to them. [Cathy]

We were taken away ... bused up about 200 miles from where we actually lived ... We were in really bad shape. So it made me feel really oppressed [prejudiced] against the government and the way they handled us. We suffered a lot of abuse ... When I first got to the boarding school we were stripped at the door and made to walk in and ... deloused. [Grace]

I think that they treated the Natives wrong ... Like they treated my mom ... wrong. I remember one day she was having one beer, right? Then they took us away. Like she is having one beer. That is all she had. They took us away. That was unfair, just because she was Native. And one beer doesn't mean you have a right to come into the house and just take us away. I think they mistreated my parents. I think that when you are Native, you are labelled right away. [Cindy]

First Nations and other women of colour were subjected to racism when they were children. Unfortunately racism did not end when they reached adulthood.

The majority of the First Nations women interviewed had experienced overt and covert racism as adults when dealing with social service agencies:

I just got a new worker and I think she's prejudiced against me because I am Native, you know ... I feel really bad when people talk bad about Native people ... Some of it is true that Native people have a lot of drinking problems and stuff. And that makes me feel bad as a person because that reflects on me, you know. That's the first impression that people have of me ... and in fact it isn't true. And I like to make myself look different from that, you know. And I want people to know that, yeah, I am Native, but I can do things too ... So I think that she is, I don't know ... Racist, yeah. Because the way she looks at me, and the way she acts around me, you know. The other worker I had was really nice. When I asked this new worker about the same things [services she had been told by her previous worker that she was eligible for] she goes, 'No that's not true.' [Sue]

I know there is no doubt, no doubt in my mind that Native Indians really get it in the neck. I mean first, they are first to lose their kids and not get them back. You know that they are the first to be whisked. [Theresa]

It was an issue. I believe if we hadn't been black they never would have come into my mother's house and taken my son. When I said to my social worker, 'How dare you go into my mother's house. You're trying to act like she didn't know how to raise my baby.' And she said, 'Well, she didn't do so good with you kids, did she.' [Greta]

A lot of people think I'm white cause I really don't look Indian, right. As soon as I show them my status card or tell them I'm Native Indian, well [snaps her fingers] their attitude changes just like this, right. [Jane]

They thought that I couldn't raise her, because of my being Native. They thought that she would probably be better off in a white home. [Grace]

Racism was prevalent in the cases of First Nations women, and women of colour who negotiated with social services. This had negative effects on both mothers and children. First Nations women in particular experienced mistrust, hostility, denial of services, surveillance, and child apprehension.

Deserving and Undeserving Women

Female welfare clients are subject to 'gender specific forms of social control' (Edwards, 1988, p. 221). The social workers' power lies in their ability to label women 'deviant' (Amir & Biniamin, 1992) and 'deserving or undeserving' (Chunn, 1995). The assessment of mothering and proper female roles is integral to welfare policy (Edwards, 1988; Maher, 1992; Maier, 1992). When women first approach the Ministry of Social Services for assistance, many are unaware of the array of interventions that this act might provoke (Gordon, 1990). Receiving assistance opens the door to surveillance by social services agencies. Women are judged according to their fitness to care for their families and their adherence to feminine virtues (Chunn, 1995; Thane, 1978). Some of the women interviewed were aware of the unwanted surveillance to which they would be subjected when applying for social assistance:

I had a lot of knowledge, and luckily I had a lot of friends that were supportive, and I didn't fall into that thing where they could have taken him away from me. Maybe somewhere deep down inside I knew to stay away from them. For me, they take babies away from people, and I've done drugs, and I've done a lot of drugs. [Morgan]

All of the mothers who were visible drug users stated that, once their drug use became known to their social workers, the relationship changed for the worse. Therefore, many hid their drug use from financial aid workers (if there are no child-protection concerns, welfare recipients are only referred to financial aid workers):

They never knew. I always, I always made sure that I hid that. [Julie]

I always kept that separate right up until ... probably the month before I asked my family to keep the kids. [Pat]

I just kept that to myself. I didn't want social services ... involved. [Cindy]

Women who use illicit drugs describe their encounters with social workers as negative experiences (Hepburn, 1993a; Maher, 1992; Taylor, 1993). Many women's illicit drug use became known to social services through health insurance claims for drug treatment, NAS diagnoses, and application for other services. Social workers have requested that illicit drug users be identified. One social worker states: 'Early identification of these people [would be] possible if it weren't for the ethical consideration of confidentiality' (Cain, 1994, p. 39). Fortunately, confidentiality still exists to some degree in relation to criminal charges. But the confidentiality of women on social assistance who use illicit drugs is rarely respected by medical and social service professionals.

Cain's (1994) interviews with social workers in B.C. reveal that 'services available to these families are numerous' but that, in the case of the illicit drug user, 'these services are seldom accepted until the effects of her addiction are blatantly threatening the safety of her children' (Cain, 1994, p. 39). Many of the women interviewed noted that, once social services became aware of their illicit drug use or legal methadone use, they were treated differently, especially when asking for other services:

And once they saw the tracks on my arms, and my hands when I was signing for my cheque, they never gave me job searches. They just gave up, just totally give up on you. [Karen]

Even with my social worker she knows about my past, and it ticks me off, 'cause she treats me like dirt. [Jane]

Oh yeah, they hate us. We don't ask them for anything. Because they say 'What did you spend your money on? Heroin?' [Marg]

She brought it up a lot, that was her main topic of conversation, my drug problem ... And at that point I was clean. [Gloria]

Revealing their illicit drug use, or having it brought to the attention of social workers, had negative consequences for the women interviewed. They were denied services and treated with less respect. They also discussed how their children were used for leverage by social workers to ensure that they had no choice but to comply with workers' demands once their illicit drug use was known. One Native Indian woman noted:

All through this, I felt like I had a gun to my head 'cause, you know, because of my circumstances with social services. 'You've got to go through treatment, you've gotta finish it. You gotta do this. If you don't finish, this is your last chance. You don't get no more chances after this.' So you're gonna have to do it or say goodbye to your kids. [Cathy]

One Native Indian mother describes the type of surveillance she experienced when her children were returned to her after a temporary child apprehension:

Then she had a court order on [me] requesting the medical history of my children, which I signed documents for. I think that she was really negative to me. Then their school history, to see how they attended school and how their progress was. Then she had a criminal record pulled on me. Done. See if I was a criminal. I signed all those. You know, it was quite stressful on me, because ... she didn't give me an easy time. Then I had a worker from parent project come down and see me for about three months and keep an eye on my home, and see how I was doing. She wrote a report about me and she said I was very oppressed [prejudiced] with the human resources. I was very sorry that I forgot to say I was oppressed [prejudiced because], of what happened to myself as a younger person. [Grace]

Single parents, poor women, and First Nations women are most at risk for social service intervention and child apprehension (Maher, 1992; Maier, 1992, Monture, 1989). In Canada, doctors and nurses often inform social services if there is suspected maternal drug use (Williams & Bruce, 1994). In this way, the providers of health care and social services collaborate in regulating and policing women (Gómez, 1994, Maher, 1992; Maier, 1992; Humphries et al., 1992; Chavkin et al., 1991). Women who use illicit drugs are reluctant to reveal their drug use, for, rather than being given support, they are punished when their drug use becomes known. In addition, when women are arrested on narcotics charges, their children are often apprehended. In this case the criminal justice system and medical and social services agencies intersect in regulating and controlling women who use illicit drugs. The interests of mother and child 'have been perceived by the state as separate, and often in conflict with each other' (Kasinsky, 1994, p. 98). Many of the women who have had contact with social services perceive social services as more problematic for them than drug laws. Some of the women stated:

Oh, social services. I slipped away from them for a long time though. It wasn't until we [participant and partner] were fighting a lot that they caught on to what was going on. And that was because it was visible. [Donna]

Oh, I think social services is worse, because they have way more power, even if I had gotten into trouble with the law, at least you get to go to court and get your case heard and have a lawyer plead your case and stuff like that. But with them, they have total power. [Greta]

It was social services that made my life a nightmare. Like I felt that they were trying to intimidate me. Like there was something that I was trying to hide. [Grace]

The criminal justice system and social services often act in tandem. Both are feared. Twelve per cent of the women interviewed stated that drug laws and social services are an equal threat to them. Two women of colour noted:

Both the same. 'Cause it was usually the cops first, cause they call social services when ... they're done with you. [Jill]

They are both heavy in my life in a sense that both of them have the ability to control what I couldn't or could do for a long time. [Mary]

However, 44 per cent of the women interviewed stated that they were more concerned about drug laws than about social service intervention. In contrast to studies that focus on poor women who use illicit drugs (Maher, 1992; Taylor, 1993), white, middle-class women who are not receiving social assistance, social service intervention seems remote. Middle- and upper-class women who were interviewed noted that the law and the fear of arrest were their primary concern. These women, having other social and economic supports available to them, had no need of social services. Their middle-class lifestyles mediated their illicit drug use, and they were not visible users:

The law, no question ... It was the law that could easily destroy people's lives ...

Recommendations could be made via the law ... I think the other thing that is important when we look at class differences is that because I came from a background where people had their own houses and had money to live, they didn't have to approach social services for money. [Debbie]

The law was more my fear. I was scared of them. I was totally afraid of them. [Sarah]

Poor women and women of colour felt the full impact of social services intervention when their illicit drug use became visible. Many of the women noted that the criminal law was regulated by due process and accessibility to lawyers, even if they were legal aid lawyers. In contrast, social workers appeared to make arbitrary decisions, had little accountability, and were able to intimidate the women, especially in relation to child custody:

The social services doesn't say to you what they mean. They will tell you in the most indirect way they can, because they're not dealing with a person when they're dealing with you, they're dealing with whatever you've done. You're not viewed as a person ... they're not going to talk to me the same way they talk to their peers. Because I'm not their peer. [Cindy]

Half the time, they don't even know what their guidelines are. You ask them to outline the situation, it is all of a sudden 'I will have to get back to you' ... Anything to avoid a direct answer to anything I want to know from her. [Pat]

You wouldn't believe it how many times I had to get on the phone and argue with those people about something. My cheque wouldn't be right. They would tell me, 'Oh you can't have this,' and I would say, 'I'm a single mom, I'm entitled to this, and I know my rights. And if you don't give me my rights, I will appeal this.' [Ellie]

The lack of guidelines, information, and due process contributed to the women's sense of vulnerability when dealing with social services. Many of the women were unaware of their rights. Those who did challenge social services discovered that knowing your rights did not always facilitate change.

Pregnancy, Birth, and Social Services

Poor women in Canada have few socio-economic supports to which to turn in relation to their caretaking role and household responsibilities (Gupta, 1995). Approaching social services often brings unwanted intervention and child apprehension. In Canada, there is little social responsibility for the care of children and for household work. Women's work in the home remains unacknowledged and unpaid, and mothers feel individually responsible for their children's care and for household break-up (Glenn, 1994; Gupta, 1995). Women who use illicit drugs are particularly fearful of approaching social service agencies for relief because of the likelihood of punitive intervention and child apprehension. The majority of fathers in this sample failed to support their children economically and emotionally; mothers had few resources to draw on outside of their own families and friends. One women of European heritage whose child was apprehended by the Ministry of Social Services sums up the difficulties facing mothers who use illicit drugs:

I think that there is a big gap in the support for women. Particulary mothers, before they get to the point where they're using drugs. I mean it takes a pretty desperate situation to make you change or slide into drug abuse. And I don't think that there is any ... help in that in-between time. You know, not totally losing it ... I have found that there was no place for me to go, knowing that I was getting into trouble with drugs. Knowing that my children as a result were going to get into trouble. [Pat]

For the majority of mothers interviewed, the care of their children was primary. The loss of children and the struggle to keep their children were at the forefront of their concerns related to illicit drug use:

Having the responsibility of raising children, I mean that is to me the most important thing, and it's a wonderful thing. But we're not really deemed even able to do that as women ... who have, you know, been drug users. Everything is taken away, everything is taken away ... I feel that I'm really lucky, I'm really lucky that I have my children. I'm lucky, but I'm still scared. [Morgan]

People die, you know. People suffer, but is that worse than having your children taken away permanently? Well, Jesus, I would probably drop off the Lions' Gate or something if they took my kids permanently. I mean that is what is keeping me going right now. It is a hard fight and I am tired of it. It is a hard fight. [Theresa]

I thought God, if I lose F., if I ever lost F., especially knowing what it feels like to lose one, it devastated me. [Jane]

If you make that commitment to be clean and stuff. And you know to really try and change your ways, you have to change everything, you know ... I don't want to get into trouble with the law any more, you know I have a baby. The last thing I ever want to do is lose him ... He's the most important thing to me. [Sue]

The mothers' fear that they might lose their children was justified, given the high child apprehension rate and frequent separation of children from mothers due to incarceration and NAS. The drudgery of household duties and the sense of sole responsibility that the women experienced were accompanied by strong bonds of love and commitment to their children. For the majority of the mothers, their children were a stabilizing force in their lives. Most important, their love for their children was accompanied by their fear of loss.

Child Apprehension

Child apprehension, whether temporary or permanent, is one tool that the welfare system wields when a mother is deemed unfit or undeserving. In Canada, child welfare laws define and legislate what is considered 'good parenting' (Pulkingham, 1994, p. 92). Social workers and the courts, through these laws, do 'intrude into the so-called "private sphere" of many families' (Pulkingham, 1994, p. 92). Poor women and women of colour – especially First Nations women – are most likely to be scrutinized and to have their children apprehended by the ministry and sent to foster care.

There is an emerging body of critical research sceptical of the foster care system (see Chavkin et al., 1991; Gupta, 1995; Hawley & Disney, 1992; Humphries et al., 1992; Maher, 1992; Monture, 1989; Noble, 1997; Report of the Aboriginal Committee, 1992). Cultural genocide and the physical, sexual, and emotional abuse of children in foster care has been emphasized. So has the punishing of mothers who do not conform to dominant ideologies of motherhood.

For poor women and women of colour, keeping the family intact is difficult because of economic and social deprivation. Of the fifty-nine children born to the twenty-eight mothers interviewed, 35 per cent were no longer in their custody. Of these, 43 per cent were permanently in the care of the ministry, and the other 57 per cent were in the permanent custody of relatives. Twenty-five per cent of the mothers had their children in temporary care of the ministry at some point in the past. Twenty-eight per cent of the mothers had been separated from their infants for long periods when their infants were in-patients at Sunny Hill Hospital's

NAS program. Of the ten children admitted to this NAS in-patient program, only three remained in the custody of their parents. In total, 36 per cent of the mothers had been separated from their children at some point because of child apprehension, relinquishing custody to relatives, or NAS in-patient care.

When children were apprehended, mothers had to appear in family court. Unlike criminal court proceedings, summary proceedings in family court are often an open forum to discuss a woman's personal life in negative terms, regardless of the successes she may have had. One Native women stated:

The thing with family court, right, they can bring up your past ... I didn't think I had a chance in hell to get them back. They're saying, 'She was a prostitute in the past, she's been busted um, you know twenty-seven times for soliciting. She's done time for it, been busted for possession. Her boyfriend is a known drug dealer and she's still involved with him and she left him (her child) with this guy, not once, but twice.' And they really made me look bad, right. And, 'Well known to the vice squad.' And I thought I don't have a chance in hell. [Cathy]

Women labelled 'deviant' and 'undeserving' by social workers were vulnerable when they appeared in family court. Other women discussed the format of family court and the likelihood of losing custody for failing to arrive in family court at the specified time, even when the mother was not informed of the hearing:

I never heard anything about it. Their excuse for that was that they couldn't find me to get in touch with me ... she was apprehended at a time that I was doing time in Oakalla ... by the time I got the letter, the court date had passed so they never made me aware of the court date. But I was in prison on that court date. I could have been transported from the prison to the court. But there was no attempt ever made, as far as I was concerned ... they send me the letter after the fact, saying 'this has all been done, because you didn't appear in court.' [Pat]

The mothers' failure to contact social services and to appear in family court was perceived as evidence of their lack of caring and unstable lifestyle.

When a mother's illicit drug use became known to social service professionals, pregnancy and birth became more complex. Medical intervention was usually initiated, and infants were often separated from the mothers and apprehended, especially after they had been labelled NAS.

When children were thought to be 'at risk,' a social worker would be assigned to the case along with the financial aid worker. An open file (social service file for child protection) would be kept until the child was no longer considered at risk. Many of the mothers noted the difference in surveillance and regulation once a social worker, rather than just a financial aid worker, was involved in their case. One Native mother stated:

Well before, they didn't even care where I was living. Until after the babies were born, right ... it's good they care about the babies and how they want them to live, right. But it was really hard for me, for them to take them away. [Jill]

Concern for the mother was secondary to the social service intervention mobilized around the children, especially once they were labelled NAS. As one of the mothers noted:

I'd just be really reluctant now to tell anybody, and you're really in a bad spot. You want to tell them because you want the medical help for your baby, but, on the other hand, by going for medical help you stand to lose your baby. [Linda]

Rather than risk losing their children, some mothers choose not to inform doctors or social workers about their illicit drug use during pregnancy:

That's why I had to lie. Absolutely. Our social worker thought an addicted [that is, an infant labelled NAS] baby is an abused baby. [Marg]

It is not unusual for social workers to perceive maternal drug use as a child-protection concern (Humphries et al., 1992; Maher, 1992; Maier, 1992). One social worker interviewed in the recent Chief Coroner's report in B.C. stated that 'perhaps we should assume that it [drug use] is always a child protection concern' (Cain, 1994, p. 39). However, illicit drug use itself does not equal poor parenting (Leeders, 1992; Hepburn, 1993a; Taylor, 1993), nor does maternal drug use have negative effects on all infants (Hepburn, 1993a, 1993b; Latchem, 1994; Myers et al., 1992; Siney, 1994, 1995). Many social factors influence maternal outcomes and parenting skills. And many social workers confuse the effects of the drug laws and poverty with the effects of illicit drug use.

Once a child has been labelled NAS, social service intervention was inevitable. The compliance of the medical community with social workers is evident in many of the hospitals in Canada, where the two work together. This ensures that children labelled NAS will be assigned a social worker:

It was the social worker at Grace [Hospital] and the head nurse who said the kid sneezed and has diarrhoea. 'We know that woman was using drugs, we'll send the baby away.' [Donna]

One Native mother described her social worker's demands upon her infant's discharge from Sunny Hill Hospital:

They were trying to get involved ... my social worker finally made ... ten contracts between me and him and it wasn't even a ministry stamp on it. It was just between him and me. And he said I had to sign it ... in order to get the baby home. The place had to be clean, drug and alcohol free environment, and that I had to be clean and sober. And I had to have a telephone in my place before the baby could come home from the hospital. What else was there? There was a lot of things there that I had to do, a support group, and that I attend AA meetings. And this was all his own idea ... And I told him to go screw himself. [Lori]

Another woman on social assistance was charged with kidnapping her own child after she ran away with her child, who was in the ministry's care, during a supervised meeting at the welfare office. In fear that her next child would also be taken by the ministry, this mother checked her son out of the hospital where he was being observed for evidence of NAS:

One [child] I took her from the welfare office, the other I checked her out of the hospital ... I had someone who was ready to pick me up, and I just walked out with her. They found me a month and a half later. They ... weren't gonna give me any chance to have her at all. And yet how could I prove I could look after her if I didn't have her, right? [Liz]

The mothers who had their children apprehended were often denied a chance to prove that they could be good parents. Mistrust of the ministry increased as mothers were denied access to their children and as it became apparent that the ministry failed to reveal its true intentions when it apprehended their children. One woman of African-American heritage stated:

The woman had really lied to my family when she came and took the baby.

Because she told my sister that the baby will only be gone for a few weeks, at the most thirty days. And we'll place him in his grandmother's care, his father's mother. And my sister said that she promised ... that within thirty days we would have my son back. But as soon as we went to court she went for a six-month order, you know she had no intention of giving him back. And so, what happened was they got their six-month order and by then I guess I had come down enough that I really had time to talk to a counsellor and stuff. And she told me, 'Maybe this is good; maybe this can be used for you to really work on yourself and you'll get to visit your son and stuff like that.' So I thought, 'Maybe this is okay.' First I went to detox, and dried up again ... I went to Aurora and I really thought that now I'm showing them that I'm really working hard. But nothing changed. I never got any more visiting time. For a year and a half. [Greta]

Informed by disease models of addiction, social workers were reluctant to believe that the mothers could cease their drug use. Many of the women discussed how this deterministic view affected them and their children:

People can't understand it, when you are screwed up. When you are not, you are not. They seem to think that somehow, like there is a residue of everything. You know, they need to see months ... of you not doing stuff before you get ... to spend time with your kids ... Like when I am screwed up, I am really screwed up and as soon as I am not, I am not. It is that simple and that quick. They say you can't shut it off and on, well I can. [Mary]

But, they didn't comprehend that you could just stop, just like that. I just stopped. She says, nobody can stop. I said, 'I beg your pardon?' I mean some of those social workers are pig-headed ... I mean as soon as they hear that you are into drugs, they don't think that you can stop. You see, when I lost him, I stopped freebasing completely. I didn't go back to it. I didn't want it. [Julie]

I heard she [social worker] phoned Sheway [a community project for women and children] yesterday. She was asking the social worker there a whole bunch of questions like she asked me the other day. 'Cause I told them I need a break from the baby and I need to take care of a whole bunch of things. And she said okay ... She asked me if the baby was born addicted and I said, 'No, he was substance free when he was born. He didn't go through any withdrawal.' And that was the first thing she asked me. And I got on the phone with her and said, 'No, that's why he is home with me.' [Lori]

The women interviewed stated that social workers were ill-informed about illicit drug use, and their misconceptions coloured their decisions. Mothers were often denied custody of their children because of their history as illicit drug users. There was little room for negotiation, and mothers stated that there was no way to 'prove' that they were capable of caring for their children once they had been labelled as illicit drug users. Separation from children often led to increased use of illicit drugs. As one mother whose children had been permanently apprehended by the ministry stated:

There should be some way to prove yourself. If you're away from your kids, it's more destructive, for them and you. [Liz]

However, as stated above, many of the women realized that there was no way to prove themselves, even if they followed all the rules and carried out all the requests of their social workers. One African-American woman described her attempt to reunite with her infant son, who had been apprehended by the ministry due to her illicit drug use. After completing a drug treatment program, she expected to gain access to her son:

I went through the program and then they expected me to come out and get a house where I would be able to bring J. Or where they could bring him to visit, and where they could check out the place and make sure it was okay. So I did that, and I was doing all the things that were required of me ... I couldn't believe there was no reward for me for doing all the stuff that I was doing. Nothing changed, and it was really hard. So, I did relapse. I was really honest about that stuff because I felt it was best to be. I didn't know that there was a kind of game you could play as long as you kept up the appearances it was okay. And that is not my nature. I'm just kind of 'what you see is what you get.' Every time I would tell her I had relapsed, she was like, 'I can't trust you.' It was getting so bad between her and I, and we just had a big blow-up and I went to the area supervisor. I just went as high as I could to say, 'Look, I hate this woman, and you better get me another social worker because I'm not responsible to what I do to her because she's got too much power over my life and I hate her guts.' They said, 'Just wait till after Christmas.'

... so after that she went to some foreign country and I got another social worker, who was really great. He was a man, and he just started the whole thing from scratch. He didn't really read all her notes and stuff. So I had a clear slate to work with him. [Greta]

Another mother of European heritage who had three children permanently apprehended by the ministry noted:

You get your kids taken away by welfare, you have a hard time living up to their expectations. Okay, with my son I was doing exactly everything that they wanted me to do to get my son, but ... [it]was never good enough. [Julie]

Other mothers had difficulty visiting their children once the children had been apprehended by the ministry. One Native mother stated:

That hurts the mum really bad. 'Cause I was totally lost for six months when they were gone ... They put them in Surrey. As if I had a car to get over there every day. And ... I had asked the worker, 'Can I see them more than one time a week?' And she says yes. But the transportation to get over there, and the lady only wanted me to go in the morning. And in the morning you have to have a two-zone, three-zone ticket to get over there, and I don't have the money for that. And they wouldn't give me the money for that. 'Cause it was over a hundred bucks for the passes. [Jill]

Both mother and infant suffered because of the social workers' prejudices, and many children were left unadopted because of the negative and often unwarranted stigma attached to prenatal drug exposure. One Native mother stated:

I told them I didn't want them going from ... home to home to home to home. Who would adopt a child the way they made her. Her medical history looked, you know. A red junkie mother. [Grace]

Approaching social services for financial assistance did not alleviate poverty; rather, women discovered that they were barely able to subsist on their monthly subsidy. One mother noted that the financial assistance she received was not enough to feed and house her children:

I mean you can't live in poverty like that for long. You either lose hope or turn to some other desperate measure, to change the situation. And [that] usually meaning getting into trouble with it. You are left with so few options and almost every one of them has a bad ending. You know ... if I could have got that financial support from welfare when I could not feed my kids for a week out of every month. When I could not even think about buying ... a luxury like cigarettes. Something too high priced and out ... of the [realm of] possibility. You know, when food, just daily nourishment was a problem; when ... you couldn't find a place that they would give you the rent money for and they were all shitty fucking dives ... and now they are giving the foster parent who has got K., they are giving her like two and a half times as much for one kid as I was getting for two. I don't see the point in all of that. What did they solve for me? Nothing, you know. [Pat]

Because of their fears regarding the negative treatment their children might receive in the care of the ministry, many of the women attempted to place their children in the care of relatives when their illicit drug use became problematic. Some of the mothers had placed their children with family when they were too young or traumatized to care for them, or because of cultural practices and expectations:

He was with one family for a while, and now he's with my aunt so I don't feel so bad ... My aunt has him, and he has six brothers. He's in my family now and now he's excellent. You'd never even know he has anything wrong with him. [Jane]

I just talked to my mom again. We are going to rotate. One week I will have her Wednesday and one week Thursday. [Mary]

He was with my family, but now I found out he is in foster care caused he wouldn't listen to my parents. Right from birth he was with my family. I didn't feel like part of it. I was just a kid and there was too much anger 'cause how I got pregnant and everything with all the rape and all those things. Ahhhhh. [Lori]

Separation and Escalated Drug Use

It is common practice in the Greater Vancouver area to remove children from their mothers' care if there is a history of illicit drug use, or if the infants have been labelled with NAS. To regain custody, mothers are expected to enter drug treatment programs and attend parenting classes in order to convince social services that they are responsible parents. However, even when mothers follow the rules, their children are not always returned. In addition, the removal of children from their mothers often has an adverse effect on the mothers' stability. When children are apprehended by the ministry the mothers' drug use often escalated, and their sense of stability ended:

Oh, I just gave up. I just thought I was no good and ... that I wasn't going to be a good mother for him ... I was so terrified about my own family background with alcoholism and that I wouldn't be able to do a good job bringing him up. I just went deeper into my addiction. [Julie]

You know, then I said, well, she is gone, and I just went right overboard. [Mary]

It was about three weeks, almost a month. It was real bad. And me not seeing them is bringing me more down. And more using I got, right. [Jill]

I didn't know there was another 200 feet to go to the ground after I lost the kids. I really did think that it would ... make my life easier. Instead, it just pulled the bottom out from underneath me. Yes. They were my only link to normality. To behave any way normal, and keeping some amount of security and stability in my life. When I lost the kids, I lost the house, the car, the jewellery, everything, and within a week, I was a street hooker, you know ... There was no reason to be anything different. I was totally, devastated. I fucked my life up. I fucked my kids' lives up. I was an unfit parent ... So ... I just dove into the drugs, of course ... to deal with all the emotional [stuff]. It doesn't matter. I could be in total hysterics and fix, and emotion gone. Just gone ... yes. So ... life pretty much became a quite a haze for me. [Pat]

When I was into drugs to cover the pain. I just want to die after losing the kids. I just want to die. [Julie]

The social stigma of losing one's child is secondary to the pain experienced. Having no legitimate way to express their pain upon the loss of their children, and few choices, many of the women increased their drug use in order to suppress their anguish. When mothers are unable to complete treatment, or fail to discontinue their illicit drug use, they fail to regain custody of their children. Thus, the initial separation of mother and infant has negative consequences with far-reaching effects in determining custody for women who use illicit drugs. Without support, many mothers begin to internalize the message that they are unfit to parent:

And I really don't know what happened but somewhere along the line I got scared. I got scared that maybe they were right and I was an unfit mother, and maybe I wasn't the best thing for my son. And so I began to sabotage myself. [Greta]

Conclusion

The underlying power struggles and race, class, and gender issues inherent in social service policy must be addressed. Currently, women who receive welfare are portrayed as an underclass of uneducated, single parents who are out of control, sexually promiscuous, and cunning (Gorlick, 1995; Martin, 1991). They have been accused of continually having children in order to stay on welfare and of regularly cheating the welfare system (Gorlick, 1995; Martin, 1991). Women receiving social assistance who are identified as illicit drug users are perceived as unfit mothers, and their children are judged to be at risk. The interests of the child and mother are often portrayed by social workers and family court judges as separate and in conflict with one another (Kasinsky, 1994).

Most social workers are white, middle-class women making decisions about other families, cultures, and lifestyles (Almonte, 1994). Often their perceptions of abuse and neglect come from their own limited and narrow ideas about the role of mothers and illicit drug use. Social workers typically had little education about cultural differences, drug use, and family formations outside of the heterosexual nuclear family. Their ignorance has negative consequences for women who come in contact with welfare agencies.

The identification of maternal drug use and the labelling of NAS have increased (Chasnoff, 1988b; Chasnoff, Burns, Schnoll, & Burns, 1985; Graham & Koren, 1991; Nulman et al., 1994; Peak & Papa, 1993; Robins & Mills, 1993; Williams & Bruce, 1994). As a result surveillance and intervention of social services in the lives of poor women and women of colour have expanded. The current attention to maternal drug use rarely supports mothers in need of economic and social assistance. Rather, it often contributes to increased drug use and instability in the family.

A social model of care is necessary for supporting women who use illicit drugs. Social workers might be included within the social model of care as both Hepburn (1990, 1993a, 1993b) and Siney (1994, 1995) have done in their programs for mothers who use illicit drugs. But, as long as social workers and social policy identify illicit drug use and behaviour outside of traditional female gender roles as deviant, women and children will suffer. What is needed is non-judgmental social and economic support, not surveillance and punishment. Finally, focusing solely on maternal drug use deflects attention from the inherent race, class, and gender bias underlying social services and society at large.

5

Drug Treatment

Drug Treatment: Experience and Usefulness

Many of the women in this study entered drug treatment in order to gain custody of their children from the ministry. Others entered treatment voluntarily in order to cease or stabilize their drug use. Although some women are able to benefit from drug treatment, a majority of the women interviewed have been subjected to inhumane and cruel treatment.

In North America, illicit drug use is predominantly viewed as a medical and/or legal problem (Alexander, 1990; Erickson, Riley, Cheung, & O'Hare, 1997; O'Hare, 1992; Peele & Brodsky, 1991). The legal model views illicit drug users as criminal, and the medical model is based on the 'addiction as disease' philosophy. Although these two models appear to be incompatible, North American drug laws and drug treatment programs have incorporated a disease/criminal model of addiction (Alexander, 1990).

Although there is no substantial evidence to support a biological or genetic mechanism that accounts for addiction, drug treatment services have adopted the philosophy that addiction is biological, progressive, and permanent (Fingarette, 1994). Drug treatment therefore requires abstinence. Treatment for licit and illicit drug use in North America has become a thriving industry, despite its low success rate (Alexander, 1990; Brecher & The Editors of *Consumer Reports*, 1972; Peele, 1989; Peele & Brodsky, 1991; Rodgers & Mitchell, 1991). Peele (1989) notes that drug treatment success rates as defined in terms of continued abstinence are less than 10 per cent. The majority of drug treatment research has focused on males, and findings have been generalized to include women (Addiction Research Foundation, 1994; Reed, 1987).

Critics of the disease-model philosophy state that both women and men have a wide range of experiences in relation to drug use (Alexander, 1990; Erickson et al., 1997; Hadaway, Beyerstein, & Yondale, 1991; O'Hare, 1992; Peele & Brodsky, 1991; Weil & Rosen, 1993). The emergence of the harm-reduction model in Europe during the 1980s has widened the debate surrounding illicit drug use and drug treatment services. Harm-reduction advocates recognize that the line separating licit and illicit drugs is culturally constructed, and has nothing to do with inherent dangerousness (O'Hare, 1992). Harm reduction recognizes that historically people have always sought ways to change consciousness through the use of drugs. Accepting this reality, harm reduction seeks to minimize the harm that drug use can cause to the individual and to society (Erickson et al., 1997; O'Hare, 1994). Rather than trying to coerce individuals to abstain from drug use, harm-reduction advocates accept drug use and focus on making drug use safer (Erickson et al., 1997; O'Hare, 1994). In addition, harm reduction attempts to search for pragmatic interventions, rather than interventions based on morality (O'Hare, 1992).

User-friendly programs such as needle exchanges and methadone maintenance exemplify the application of the philosophy of harm reduction. The harm-reduction movement offers a serious counterbalance to the supremacy of the disease model of addiction, and harm reduction is growing in popularity in North America.

A person's relationship to drugs may be positive or negative, and this may shift according to personal expectations and environmental influences – set and setting (Weil & Rosen, 1993; Zinberg & Harding, 1979). Harm-reduction advocates agree that drug use ranges from positive experiences to problematic ones; therefore, abstinence is unnecessary and unrealistic for many drug users. Harm reduction does not reject abstinence. Rather, it includes abstinence in a wide range of options for the drug users.

Most people who use alcohol or other drugs develop healthy relationships with their drugs of choice and are able to use them recreationally without fear of escalating or problematic use. However, a small minority of drug users, at certain times, do develop problematic relationships with drugs, and this can be very frightening. One middle-class woman in her late forties described her relationship with drugs:

I am stuffing myself ... like somebody stuffing themselves with food. When it comes to drugs, alcohol and cigarettes, it's insatiable ... I have to keep doing it, doing it and doing it. And doing ... it fills it up. It fills up ... I am terrified to go out. I'm terrified to stop. Just like in a snow storm. I was thinking about this. In snow storms, there is a fucking blizzard out, it's big time. It's dangerous. Okay, I say my life is very dangerous. In a snow storm, if you keep going, you can't see, you might have an accident ... But, if you stop, somebody can hit you from behind. I mean it is just as fucking dangerous. You have got to keep going. So, what do you do in a snow storm? You don't stop. You keep going because the worst thing to do is stop ... It is just like ... like I'm living in a snow storm, I feel like I'm fucking driven. [Judy]

It would be misleading to omit the small percentage of drug users who find their drug use problematic and painful. The majority of the women interviewed had experienced problematic and negative drug use. Problematic drug use can be devastating to both the individual and her family. Any person raised in a family where problematic addiction existed will attest to the pain witnessed and experienced.

The image of the problematic drug user has been popularized by the media in North America (Alexander, 1990; Erickson et al., 1987; Waldorf, Reinarman, & Murphy, 1991). However, rather than contributing to our understanding of drug use, the stereotype presented by the media has limited our understanding. Not all women feel driven by their drug use, even when they are dependent on illicit drugs. Nor are patterns of drug use static. The reasons why people use drugs in a dependent and addictive manner are complex and individual. Where one woman may trace her addiction to familial abuse, another may have had a happy home life. Not all addiction[1] is negative and problematic. Many of the women interviewed were able to normalize their lives and stabilize their drug use even though they were physiologically addicted.

Both compulsory and voluntary drug treatment are often offered to people who use drugs. The components of drug treatment may include detox, abstinence, counselling, residential treatment, and drug maintenance. Traditionally, in North America, drug treatment embraces a disease model. Abstinence and relapse prevention are primary. The majority of the women interviewed for this study had participated in some form of drug treatment, ranging from individual counselling to Alcoholics Anonymous (AA), detox, methadone maintenance, and residential drug treatment. Many of the women interviewed had to participate in drug treatment programs in order to regain custody of their children. Others voluntarily entered treatment programs in order to cease their illicit drug use. Some entered drug treatment through probation orders.

In response to the question 'Do you think alcohol and drug treatment

TABLE 5.1
Interviewees Who Found Alcohol and Drug Treatment Effective

Total Sample: 28	N	%
Treatment was effective	5	18
Treatment was not effective	14	50
Treatment might be effective if treatment policy changed radically	9	32

is effective?' the women interviewed were quite adamant about drug treatment reform (see table 5.1). When asked whether drug and alcohol treatment is effective, 18 per cent (5) of the women said yes, 50 per cent (14) said no, and 32 per cent (9) thought drug treatment might be effective if treatment policy changed radically (see table 5.1). All of the women interviewed gave suggestions for drug treatment reform, and many gave descriptive examples of their own experiences in drug treatment. Few believed in the disease model of addiction, and even fewer accepted the philosophy of AA and NA (Narcotics Anonymous). A wide range of drug maintenance and treatment options were discussed, as was the view that acceptance of drug use, rather than treatment, was necessary.

Some of the women interviewed noted that drug treatment and AA had been useful to them:

Yeah, I think it works. 'Cause when I did make that decision I can still draw on a lot of the information I got there. [Greta]

If I didn't have AA I would be totally using, or drinking or going crazy. [Ellie]

However, the majority of the women interviewed had negative experiences in relation to drug treatment based on the disease model, which is used in the AA philosophy. Rigid policy and inhumane practices left many of the women sceptical of the overall benefit of drug treatment. One woman noted that her time in drug treatment was similar to 'being in jail' [Cathy]. Another woman stated:

I think the way treatment was set up here, and still today, is horrible. [Hope]

Residential drug treatment is one option for drug users, and many women who are mothers are directed to residential drug treatment centres as a requirement for receiving access to their children following child apprehension by the Ministry of Social Services. The women interviewed described residential drug treatment:

Treatment was very dehumanizing. There was no understanding of the issues involved. Everyone was treated the same. I was in Maple Ridge, Brannon Lake. Brannon Lake was a boot camp. What a joke. But most of all it was completely ineffective for me and actually harmful. It's difficult to be treated like a criminal, like a child too, when you're not ... This whole concept of tough love and behavioural modification is such bullshit. People's needs are very different, and people's motivations and actions are different. There is no such thing as tough love. Love has to do with acceptance, not coercive confrontation. [Hope]

All of those programs ... they're so precarious most of the time and if you fuck up once you're out. Even if you don't fuck up, if your attitude is not right. If they don't like ... your idea for your future lifestyle. You know, if they don't like your schooling program or whatever it is. If it doesn't fit into their rigid idea of what is normal, then they withdraw the support. Or they totally go out of their way to get you arrested or get you ... you know, fucked up with the law or back in prison or stuff. And just undermining whatever efforts that you are making. They may not be a hundred per cent efforts. Maybe you are still struggling with yourself to really ... really do this a hundred per cent, but ... I think that as long as you are struggling to any degree, you deserve the sanctuary to do it in. [Pat]

For many of the women, being away from their family and friends was especially difficult. Many drug treatment programs discourage participants from associating with their family. One Native mother stated:

The counsellors ... I didn't get off with her at all ... you know, but I opened up to her ... She told me, 'Oh well, you can't go to your house.' And I said, 'What do you mean I can't go to my house.' And she said, 'Well you have free time this weekend but you're not allowed to go to your house, cause it's a high risk area, you don't know if your boyfriend is gonna be there.' [Cathy]

Although family and friends are perceived by workers as risk factors for participants in drug treatment, families and friends can offer support which is beneficial (Taylor, 1993). Many ex-users have been able to maintain contact with their families and friends regardless of their continued drug use. One professional woman from a working-class background stated:

Many of the members of my family have problems with addiction and drug dependence. I'm sure this is quite common. At first, because all of the counsellors and drug treatment and books on addiction state that you have to stay away from this dysfunctional system, I distanced myself from my family. But, you know, this was a huge mistake. My family may have addiction problems, but they are my family and I love them, too. So now I see them. I negotiate and renegotiate with myself how much. And if I feel unsafe about my own sobriety, well I know how to take care of that now without feeling like I have to banish my family from my life. It's a terrible thing to tell people they can't be with their family or friends. What a lonely, alienating thing to do to people. Just when you need support, they take it from you. It's such a straight, white, middle-class conception to think that you can just cut your family off like that. [Hope]

The women who participated in residential drug treatment were often separated from their own children, as well from other family members. Few residential drug programs have facilities for children, and as Rosenbaum and Murphy (1987) note, mothers are reluctant to leave their children behind. Many women have no one to care for their children while they are in residential treatment. Many of the mothers discussed how social workers forced them to enter drug treatment and to stay in it when they wished to leave. When mothers have no childcare options while they attend drug treatment, children become temporary wards of the court if they are placed voluntarily in foster care. As discussed by Taylor (1993), many mothers believed that if they did not complete their drug treatment program successfully their children would be taken from them permanently. One mother who is currently a full-time student stated:

I felt that I needed help and I went to social services and they recommended me to a place downtown, I think it was on Hastings. And they said, I could go, they'd get me into a place right away. And I would stay there for three weeks and go on a methadone withdrawal. And that was all part of it and they took my son into a foster care home. And then I went and as soon as I got there they told me there wasn't going to be any methadone withdrawal, it was gonna be, you know, a cold turkey withdrawal. And this was after they already had my child, and there was nothing I could do. You know, I couldn't just go home. The only thing they did was help me with the childcare so I could deal with the problems I was having. But I wasn't comfortable with that because they basically tricked me into doing that. I thought that was bizarre and I was real angry. [Morgan]

When mothers have a history of drug use, or if their infant is labelled

NAS at birth, they may be forced or coerced into treatment in order to gain access to their infants. Several mothers on social assistance described their admittance to drug treatment after the birth of their children:

Yeah, about two days after my son was born I was bounced to detox. It was my decision, but I didn't really want to. I had to because the social services was getting involved with it, with him. They were trying to apprehend him ... And I didn't see him for about ten days after that. [Lori]

Actually, when I got out of Grace Hospital I was going to stay in Homestead because I was going into their program. But they kicked me out because they said that I needed to leave my baby where he was and just focus on their program. And they said that because their program wasn't a priority over my son, that I would have to leave. I said to them, 'Are you serious? After being told my son could have a seizure and do all this stuff, you expect me to forget about that and focus on this program?' And that was expected. [Greta]

Drug treatment was difficult for some of the mothers who were able to bring their children, for they were restricted in caring for them. The drug treatment program was deemed by drug workers to be more important than the infant. Mothers were not able to care for their children as they felt necessary. One Native mother noted:

I didn't like it because they wouldn't let me breast-feed either. That pissed me right off ... They wouldn't let me breast-feed and I had to get the doctor to phone and by that time he was already using formula. The only time he cried was when he was hungry, right. Well um, they had, they had a special agency where they came in, these ladies, and watched the kids. They didn't allow it, right. But now they do because I just couldn't stop breast-feeding in the middle of everything and that's what I would have had to do. Because you can't be late for class, because you earn like three demerits. Yeah, yeah, if you were even like three minutes late, because I was feeding my kid, you know. You get demerits.

So I ended up being on reflections for almost the whole time I was there ... Reflections means you're not allowed to make any phone calls. You're not allowed to receive any phone calls; you're not allowed to leave there ... I spent a lot of time on reflections. It sort of defeated itself in a way, too, because I felt like I couldn't share totally of myself. 'Cause some of the things I didn't agree with. I just, I just knew I had to use a lot of 'I' statements because that's what they like to hear, and ah ... Well I never read whole studies but, you know, like, 'I am feeling angry because, you know.' You know you had to express your anger in certain ways. [Cathy]

The mothers' wish to care for their children often led to conflict with staff, and consequently their experiences of residential drug treatment was negative and often incomplete, for many of the mothers were unable to finish the program.

In addition to conflicts regarding mothering, many of the mothers experienced religious and racial conflicts while in treatment:

Not many Native women in there to begin with. And they really pushed on the God th ing too. They say they don't but they do. They have Bible study and you had to go to church. [Cathy]

During the interview period Vancouver had only two residential drug treatment centres that would accept children. As of fall 1995, there are no residential treatment centres in Vancouver that will accept children. In the Lower Mainland, only one residential treatment centre (in Abbotsford) will accept mothers and children and it has a lengthy waiting list. Mothers have limited options for treatment and limited chances of regaining access to and custody of their children. Private drug treatment is not a viable for poor women, and long waiting lists exist for the few government-funded treatment centres available to them.

One mother from an upper-middle-class background described how detox occurred in her family:

I think the other thing that is important when we look at class differences ... There was detoxing that happened in our house ... a chronic detoxing. But I didn't understand ... it was never defined to me as such, because we didn't have to take that person and put them into the Salvation Army detox, or what have you. My family would put them in the basement ... They would go through detoxing in our basement but we were forbidden to go down there and they never came up and took food with us, and I knew that there was some mysterious thing going on in the basement ... And it was such a bizarre thing. But it was never ever talked about in its true name ... so it was never talked about. This person is down in the basement withdrawing and having DTs from alcoholism. Never, never would that stuff be discussed. [Debbie]

Options available to mothers who use drugs are limited through differential access to drug treatment and social and economic support, and the stigma attached to poor mothers who are identified by social services as known drug users. Once a woman enters a drug treatment centre, social services become aware of her drug use either through the initial approval or later through medical reimbursement. One professional woman described her past encounters with social services after she attended Maple Ridge, a residential drug treatment program:

> I found that social services treated me really harshly ... They knew, you know, [that she had been in drug treatment] it was on my file. Other people got a bus pass but I didn't ... they had all that information [about drug treatment], it was right there. And the thing is, the woman I was seeing was talking about it more than she was talking about anything else. [Gloria]

Although many social workers insist on drug treatment for their female clients (Cain, 1994), the stigma attached to this action makes it difficult for woman once they complete the program. Upon entering a drug treatment program, poor women who have been able to conceal their illicit drug use from social services are subsequently identified and stigmatized.

Methadone: A Maintenance Program

Not all illicit drug users enter drug treatment in order to withdraw or abstain from drugs. A minority of long-term users opt for maintenance programs. In British Columbia, methadone maintenance is one option for users who have become addicted to opiate derivatives. Patients are eligible for methadone maintenance only after they have proved that other drug treatment has failed, that they have been addicts for many years, and that they will comply with the rules responsibly (Alexander, Beyerstein, & MacInnes, 1987). Methadone maintenance allows legal, unadulterated, orally administered methadone to be prescribed to some people addicted to narcotics. Methadone maintenance programs emerged in the 1960s in the United States. Dole and Nyswander were the first doctors to experiment with methadone maintenance, and they later established the first methadone clinics in the United States (Dole, 1987). It has been demonstrated that methadone maintenance allows people to lead a normal life, rather than a criminal life (Alexander, 1990; Alexander et al., 1987; Brecher & The Editors of *Consumer Reports*, 1972; Dole & Nyswander, 1965; Knight et al., 1996; Wijngaart, 1991). In addition, oral methadone maintenance allows people to stop using needles, which reduces the incidence of infections such as hepatitis and HIV.

The methadone program in B.C. has been controversial and subject to Ministry of Health policy changes since its establishment in 1963. When methadone maintenance in B.C. was first established, it was described as a lifetime program for patients. Unfortunately, the early promises were never carried out, and methadone maintenance is not a secure lifetime program. Rather, methadone patients in B.C. are often subject to cruel experimentation, regulation, and drastic shifts in policy.

Currently, both private doctors and government clinics provide prescriptions to patients. All methadone patients must be federally approved and registered in order to receive methadone, and physicians must be federally licensed to prescribe it. Both private doctors and government clinics are regulated by the Federal Bureau of Dangerous Drugs, the B.C. Medical Association, and the police (Alexander, 1990).

The B.C. Ministry of Health has regularly tried to limit the practice of private physicians in relation to prescribing methadone. The ministry claims that private physicians overprescribe and profit from prescribing methadone, and that legal methadone is diverted and sold on the street (Alexander et al., 1987). However, Alexander, Beyerstein, and MacInnes (1987) state that there are no data to support the ministry's claims.

Drug testing and daily pick-up of methadone prescriptions is routine, though in the past some private doctors in B.C. have allowed their older, more stable methadone patients to pick up less often. Although methadone maintenance offers a break from the illegal activities associated with illicit drug use and the *possibility* of a more stable and normal life, most drug users perceive it as a last resort:

Oh shit! I did everything in God's green earth to avoid going on methadone. I did not want my name in Ottawa. [Theresa]

I don't think people want to go on methadone, because, number one, they know they're going to be given a low dosage; number two, the pressure now is to get off methadone. There's so much pressure to lower your dosage and get off it. And it's harder to get off of than heroin, so you get a street addict who's getting high-quality, low-cost heroin and ... first of all, most people don't want to go on methadone. It's like admitting defeat to yourself. You really are. You're saying, 'Look, I've tried to quit ... I can't quit, I can't beat it.' ... I don't care who they are, nobody likes to do that. And then you get a program that's got rules that basically penalize people for going on methadone. [Linda]

Twenty-five per cent of the women interviewed were on legal methadone, and 36 per cent had been on methadone maintenance and methadone withdrawal programs in the past (see table 5.2).

TABLE 5.2
Legal Methadone Use

Total Sample: 28	N	%
Never prescribed legal methadone	11	39
On legal methadone at the time of the interview	7	25
On legal methadone in the past	10	35

All of the women who had been on methadone maintenance stated that methadone was a much harsher drug than heroin in terms of short- and long-term effects and longer withdrawal period:

The only alternative people are given is methadone and methadone is a really tough one because that is like the hardest habit to kick. God only knows what it does because it's not organic. Your bones, ugh ... They wouldn't legalize something more natural for your body or easier to withdraw from. It's got to be this thing that is so heavy duty. Poison. It was invented by the Nazis ... we owe it all to the Nazi scientists. [Gloria]

Like the methadone patients studied by Rosenbaum and Murphy (1987) in the San Francisco Bay area, the women interviewed expressed a dislike for the effects of methadone and worried about the harm it could cause them long-term. In addition, many researchers have noted that drug treatment services fail to address the needs of women (Addiction Research Foundation, 1994; Ashbrook & Solley, 1979; Bepko, 1991; Ettorre, 1992; Kasl, 1992; MacKinnon, 1991; Mondanaro, 1989; Reed, 1987; Rosenbaum, 1981; Rosenbaum & Murphy, 1987; Taylor, 1993)

The Program

Becoming a patient on methadone maintenance requires strict adherence to many rules, and not every narcotics user is accepted. Illicit drug users who cannot show needle marks are rarely considered for methadone treatment programs. One long-term legal methadone patient noted:

Now, there was somebody who was addicted to smoking heroin, they tried to get on methadone, they couldn't get off and they're dead now. They couldn't get on the program 'cause they had no needle marks. [Linda]

Needle marks, long-term addiction, several drug treatment attempts, and compliance and responsibility are the usual requirements for entering a treatment program. Patients are regularly tested for drugs that are not approved and legally prescribed by their methadone physician. They must provide urine samples, and urine screening is often supervised by a staff member. To be explicit, this means that patients must urinate on demand, often in full view of a drug worker. One professional woman stated:

When I was in treatment it was very similar to jail. You were denied privileges. You had to pee every day in front of a worker who was just like a guard. If you couldn't pee you didn't get your methadone. And I couldn't pee with this person staring at me, so it was a real problem. [Hope]

Expulsion from the program follows if a patient is unable to provide a urine sample or continues to show dirty screens (meaning that the urine test is positive for drugs other than methadone) or is unable to follow the many other rules. Pick-up times for prescriptions and counselling are often rigid, and maximum daily doses in British Columbia are eighty milligrans of methadone (Alexander et al., 1987). Private doctors appear to be more flexible with their patients than are clinic doctors; however, this is not consistent.   '

One woman currently on welfare assistance described her early encounter with the program when methadone maintenance was perceived as a lifetime program for patients:

I went into the Narcotic Foundation, spoke to the doctor. In those years they really encouraged you to go on methadone, and they sat you down and said, 'Look you've tried this several times, you've tried withdrawal, this is methadone maintenance. In all probability it's a lifetime program. But we believe that there's certain people that the program will help, and obviously, you know, you're in that category. So give it a try.' So, I went on it. [Linda]

Some of the long-term methadone patients spoke about their experiences in relation to diminishing methadone doses, trust, and the effectiveness of the current methadone program:

I recall a doctor asking me, could I still feel my fixes, because the idea in methadone maintenance was to block heroin. Now, unfortunately they've got away from this idea in the last few years and this has really affected ... you know, how the program works. Anyway, I was on, I think, 140 milligrams ... Anyway in the last couple of years, now they've made a maximum of eighty and at the same time while they've diminished the dosage and coupled with the fact that there's high-quality heroin on the street ... I see people that have done well on methadone quitting the program. [Linda]

Oh, God. There is so much, you know, that I could say. All the years that I've been on the program and all the changes that they have thrown at us ... they talked about trust and they lied to us. But, we never lied to the extent that they lied to us. I mean, to the point of where we were guinea pigs ... I mean, what they were doing, was testing our ... what do you call it, our points ... to what point ... how far could they push us until we, you know, got angry. You know, how far could they go ... you know? Like ... I was on 80 mg ... how far can they push me down before I would react and what kind of reaction could they get from me? [Evelyn]

The original methadone programs envisioned by Dole and Noorlander in the 1960s advocated methadone doses that were high enough to block the heroin effect and withdrawal symptoms (Dole, 1987). The Ministry of Health guidelines dictate a maximum of eighty milligrams of methadone daily, which is too low for many patients.

The structure of methadone programs, whether they take place in clinics or are run by private doctors (following guidelines by the Ministry of Health), hinder patient compliance. One woman described her initial visit to the methadone clinic in Vancouver in 1980 when she was on welfare:

I was so sick, because usually when you decide to go on methadone, you are pretty desperate. This doctor, he keeps asking me how I made my money to buy drugs, during my visit with him to see if I was eligible for the program. I told him I sold drugs. But he keeps insisting, 'Well, how do you really make your money?' Finally, I realize he is implying that I am prostituting, and finally I realize if I don't just agree this is what I do, I'm probably not going to get on the program. Because you see he had a set idea of who I was, and by trying to state otherwise I appeared to be lying and not complying with the program. So I just let him think what he wanted to because I needed to get on the program. But, you know, I only lasted about four weeks because I couldn't follow all the rules. [Hope]

Many of the women interviewed described how they were stereotyped as 'bad' women, and treated as less than their male counterparts. The sexism they encountered and the humiliation they experienced in complying with many of the rules deterred many women from staying on the program. The rules often made living a normal life difficult for the women on methadone. Another professional woman described her experience at a methadone clinic:

Well, the methadone clinic in X, as far as I am concerned, is a nightmare from hell. It is just ... There is nothing good about the program. The only good thing is that you are ... you get methadone, So uh ... you are allowed to carry on your life, but no ... the way that people are treated, is ... you are treated like objects ... Okay, you have to go there every day between 7 and 10 [a.m.]. I didn't even mind that so much when I am in town. Then you have to go to a group meeting between 8:30 and 10:00 on Tuesday or Thursday morning. It didn't matter if you were working or what, you had to be there. And ... you were allowed to have one four-day carry every three months only, so that is four times a year. They had to be every three months. I said that it wouldn't even be so bad if it was four a year and you could choose when you needed them, no.

So, ultimately, it made it impossible for me to live a normal life. My parents are older, living in X. I like to visit them. Never mind any other holidays. Then in my employment, I was requested to go to work shops and stuff outside of the city and I wasn't allowed to do it, unless of course it fell within the three-month period of time. If I had to teach class at 8:30 in the morning, too bad. I mean I was expected to miss it to go to this group meeting which was just a joke to begin with. [Diane]

Although most of the clinics insist on daily pick-up, some private physicians have allowed patients to come less often. One woman who was a full-time student described her experience with a private doctor:

It is ... I mean now, it is three days a week. How in God's name am I going to go to anything but university when I have to get somewhere three days a week? Yes, I have to give a urine sample, almost daily ... [Now] I go to my doctor's once a week, but his is not a clinic setting. I'm his only patient as far as I know. I go there and then twice a week I pick up the methadone, so that is ... he considers that to be ... that works out to three times a week. Right now, that is about the average I go, about three times a week. Is that what you found? [Theresa]

The wide range of policy, from daily pick-up and supervised drug testing to pick-up three times a week and unsupervised drug testing, often appears arbitrary. There were no rewards for compliance and successful long-term maintenance. Long-term patients were treated the same as newcomers. The women noted:

Well, the sad thing is ... it is not even twenty years ... I mean the people that have been on for twenty years, and I know people that have been on ... they have just as hard a time now, as if they were brand-new addicts ... They have to leave all these urine samples the same as everybody else. It is awful. It is just totally awful. You know, the situation. [Theresa]

I can relate to a little bit of rigidity at the beginning, when people come on. I can relate to that. But, it doesn't change. No matter how long you are there and no matter how long you behave, it doesn't matter, you are treated the same. It interferes with your employment, they make it impossible for you to live a normal life. Absolutely impossible. [Diane]

Maintaining a normal lifestyle was difficult, given the rigid structure of methadone maintenance, and the women found the rules humiliating. One middle-class woman in her late forties described being subjected to body searches at the methadone clinic she now attends outside of B.C., and the humiliation she experiences now in contrast to earlier treatment by a private doctor in Vancouver:

Oh, yes. Every day you have to go in there and you have to ... you are subjected to body searches. The nurses, I guess ... they are a lot younger than me, they are twenty years younger than me. I find it very ... I find them condescending. I just find it's very undignified. For a woman of my age and because I am a proud woman. I find the whole process undignified. And, and ... I just find it hard to even talk about it, Susan, because all of a sudden I feel I'm gonna burst into tears. I hate the whole indignity of it. I just hate it. But, I keep trying to say to myself to pretend it is insulin that you are going to get. Pretend it is insulin. But, it isn't and I know in my mind that [it] isn't that. It is just very undignified the way you're treated like a kid. Like a juvenile delinquent. When I was in Vancouver, it never used to hurt me as much. Whether it has something to do with my age difference, but it just didn't torment me emotionally as much going in once a week. [Judy]

Being able to pick up methadone once a week allowed the women to stabilize, to maintain jobs, and to centre on activities other than their addiction to methadone. Fewer pick-ups a week also allowed the women to escape the implementation of humiliating rules attached to obtaining their methadone. The women believed that the rules they had to follow while on methadone maintenance discouraged stability. They explained:

You just can't work and it makes it really difficult. In other words, all the ... they've implemented rules that basically, to me they're saying, well, we'll give you metha-done but we're going to make your lifestyle inconvenient, we're going to discour-age you so you get off methadone ... and it's not realistic. [Linda]

When I was on ... a methadone program and having to go every day and go to the bathroom with the door open and drink my little methadone there and never be able to take a holiday and never be able to carry for even two or three days to get away, like normal people ... they encourage you to stay in the same rut that you are in. [Carol]

As early as 1981 Rosenbaum noted that social control was an aspect of methadone programs. Although the women interviewed on methadone maintenance were hoping to normalize their life and to participate in other activities unrelated to their narcotic addiction, the rigid structure of most methadone maintenance programs made this impossible.

Overall, rigid treatment programs can be harmful to patients, and expensive. There is substantial evidence that compulsory counselling, rigidity, and drug testing are not effective, and have no positive effect either for the patient or for program success (Alexander, 1990; Alex-ander et al., 1987; Noorlander, 1987; Wijngaart, 1991). In the Nether-lands, drug testing is discouraged and methadone patients are allowed to top up their methadone with other drugs (Wijngaart, 1991). The goal of 'methadone maintenance care' in the Netherlands is harm reduction. Offering education and prevention to drug users takes priority over puni-tive rules that may discourage narcotics users from entering programs (Wijngaart, 1991).

The women interviewed also felt restricted in their search for a doctor to prescribe methadone. One low-income woman explained:

I actually would like to look for another doctor, because ... he doesn't like us and he is very obvious about that too. He has got all these little punishment things. You know, if you can't ... if you can't give a sample [urine sample] when he asks for it, he takes ten milligrams off your prescription. [Evelyn]

Very few private doctors are federally licensed and government clinics are usually more repressive than programs run by private physicians. When women and men are unable to urinate on demand for drug testing, they are punished by having their methadone dosage lowered.

The women interviewed described the sexist attitude of many of the doctors who prescribed methadone. One woman noted how she was continually ignored by doctors during her twenty years on methadone. Instead of speaking to her directly, the doctor always addressed her husband, D.:

When they would call us in, and that was a private doctor, if they wanted to tell us about a mandate, 'Oh, D., will you come here for a minute?' Never once did they speak to me. Together with D., or if D. was in the washroom, it would be, 'Where's D.?' Blatant, blatant, blatant. Of all the years, of almost twenty-five years of being on methadone. [Marg]

Because many of the doctors who prescribed methadone held sexist attitudes about the proper role of women, as Reed (1987) notes, it is difficult for women to communicate their needs to doctors and treatment staff.

Other women noted that some doctors were uneducated about methadone and, similiar to Rosenbaum and Murphy's (1987) findings, the women suffered when they had health problems. One common misconception doctors had was that the women did not experience pain when they were on methadone. This has serious consequences, especially during labour and birth. One woman in her early fifties stated:

Too often you go into a doctor, 'Oh you're on methadone, you shouldn't feel any pain.' I mean, it's so ridiculous. [Linda]

Although the majority of the women who had participated in methadone programs were negative about their experience, those few who were able to find less rigid private physicians were optimistic about the changes that had occurred in their lives and the opportunities for employment and stability that were now available to them. One middle-class woman described her difficulty dealing with the drug scene and the criminal overtones that government clinics promote:

Another thing is that you are ... when you are down in the goddamn clinics, you are constantly subjected to people who aren't necessarily in the same space that you are. They love to talk about it, that's their life. It is their lover. It is their companion, drugs are. If you are trying to get away from that, it is really hard, because of course, sometimes, who you hang out with, you become one of. So, when everybody is talking drugs and criminal, you end up being the same. Where if you pop in once a week, you're in and out of there ... Like in Vancouver, I was there for what ... seven years and I went to the same doctor. I never got to know one patient. Not one, because ... I was in and out. [Judy]

In contrast to the clinic experience, another middle-class woman described her experience with a private doctor as more beneficial to stability:

If you go to the doctor once a week or twice a week ... that doesn't become the focal point of your life any more. Your life moves on to other things. You are not kept in that ... that little world of, sort of, that underworld. You move out from there. I am highly successful now and part of it is because I got on a methadone program, got on with a doctor who ... had more of a philosophy, ... from the European nation, that ... I was not a criminal. This was more of medical problem and that it would be treated as a medical problem. And that I was a person that was not stupid and could make decisions for myself ... my husband and I are perfect examples of how much better we have done, since we have been allowed to do that. [Carol]

As shown in the qualitative study of Knight et al. (1996) on women who had been on subsidized methadone maintenance treatment in the United States, women can stabilize and decrease illicit activity and increase employment and educational goals when methadone is affordable and available.

The women interviewed were very adamant that drug use and addiction were not a criminal problem. However, as long as specific drugs were criminalized, one professional woman concluded:

Well, I think as long as it is against the law, illegal ... I think that private doctors are really the only answer, unless clinics were run in a different way than they are now. [Diane]

Given the current legal status of their drugs of choice, the women favoured a medical model, in consultation with private doctors.

The women, especially long-term methadone patients, were informed about the many controversies surrounding private physicians prescribing methadone in B.C. One low-income woman stated:

I ... think that physicians who prescribe to users are definitely seen as drug pushers. Y'know, I think that other doctors, even when they've read literature, have absolutely no understanding of the whole complexity of what that's all about and they perceive them as these drug pushers and really do pressure them to lower [dosages] and to have few patients. If they see them getting a lot of patients they start thinking all these weird things, like, oh yeah, easy to come in and give them a prescription and they can bill ... they just have no idea how complex it is. [Linda]

Methadone and Alternatives

Many of the women offered suggestions for methadone maintenance reform. Several women noted that methadone maintenance programs were inflexible, for patients had to take their methadone every day, regardless of need. One professional woman stated:

All the methadone treatment places you get your drug every day. So there is no support for the occasional user, the Sunday user. Most users are concerned with the supply of their drug. Where will it come from next? Will there be enough? Will it be available to me if I quit? It keeps people on the program because there is no experimenting, not on the client, but allowing them to try using once a week, twice a week, going up to every day when they want to, or down to once a week again with no penalty attached. Or someone who feels they could stabilize at a few heroin cigarettes every Sunday. I think if I had a choice, it's difficult to say this because we don't have a choice. But I would be, as an older person, happier to have that available to me, occasional use of drugs like opium and heroin. I don't use at all, because I don't want to re-enter that illegal scene or place myself in jeopardy of AIDS, or hep, abscesses, all those things that the black market fosters ... I think a lot of people stay on maintenance because they're afraid that if they cut back, or suggest less methadone a day, the treatment centre or doctor will see it as a failure if they ask for more. Or will just deny them access to more. So it creates this constant anxiety for users going into treatment. It's an all-or-nothing situation. And that is unrealistic and creates longing, anxiety, and eventually leads to increased use. [Hope]

The current practice of only daily maintenance options was perceived as contributing to further addiction rather than experimentation with occasional drug use and shifts in use.

Another common suggestion by the women interviewed was the use of methadone patients on decision-making boards that would guide methadone programs and ministry decisions. One long-term methadone patient stated:

Well, one change is that they have to ... they have to get somebody in there that, you know, who is not biased. You know, the whole committee ... who sets up the regulations and everything ... they have got people in there who do not like the program ... don't believe in the program, they don't like it, they wish, you know, it didn't exist. These are the people who are supposed to be on our side, kind of. Like they are supposed to be there to kind of help us. Of course they are not helping us ... what I would like to see is ... more input from ... like with R. or B., and M., myself, you know, some input into this committee so that we can say, you know, look ... we don't feel that is right, but we are not asked a thing. You know, out of all the knowledge that I think that I have ... which has been a lot of years. You know, I think that I could contribute a lot of information. [Evelyn]

Many of the women interviewed felt that their experience as long-term methadone patients would be useful, and would contribute to more efficient and humane programs. McDermott and McBride (1993) discuss how successful coalitions between drug users and drug workers can be. The women noted that drug testing, monitoring and daily visits are expensive. Although they stated that not all drug users will stabilize, they felt the majority would, given the opportunity:

I'd like to see users treated as mature adults. No piss tests, no penalties, no dogma, no new religion that you have to adopt. I think professionals in treatment are more fucked up than their clients. Though I'm not 100 per cent sure about reformed addicts, some of them are as bad. But I'd like to see treatment as user-friendly, with ex-addicts and addicts on the board so things don't get out of hand. If people feel they need treatment. [Hope]

One woman noted that it would be beneficial to include methadone patients on boards for often many of the narcotic users were aware of who the long-term users were. One long-term methadone patient stated that this would eliminate new users from being admitted to the program when other options had not been tried:

But, I think that in terms of clinics that, that clinics should have boards which have addicts on them, even addicts that are presently using the clinic, and that they should be involved with the other people who are running the clinic ... One of the reasons that a lot of the wrong people got on methadone, because all of the addicts knew who this person was and that they should not be getting methadone. But the people that are running didn't because they didn't have any experience in that area. [Carol]

Drug Use, Withdrawal, and Cessation

Drug Withdrawal

Although some long-term illicit drug users, and especially narcotics users, opted for methadone maintenance, many had tried to withdraw completely from drug use several times. Some of the women interviewed were successful in withdrawing and remaining abstinent; others have used occasionally since withdrawing. Some were unable to stop using. Almost all of the woman had withdrawn from drugs at home. Some of these attempts were more successful than others. The women noted that withdrawal at a drug treatment centre was not always a viable option:

No, I just did it on my own. I've never been to treatment. [Sue]

No, I always did it myself. [Marg]

I didn't use any of that. I have no idea. It never seems all that effective to me. [Janet]

Withdrawing from heroin is less difficult than withdrawing from methadone, and many of the woman felt that they lost their autonomy when trying to withdraw from methadone. Withdrawing as a methadone patient often meant that the physician, rather than the woman, controlled the dose. Several women described methadone withdrawal:

I wanted to be told, I wanted control of my destiny. I mean, I am not a kid here. It was ... another part of the whole humiliating process. I said, 'Look, I am a middle-aged woman. I want control of my own destiny, I want to know what doses that I am on.' Well, they say, 'Why does it mean anything to you?' [Judy]

It took me a month to decide to do it, because I went through the workers and I said, 'Look, this is my withdrawal, you know. When I say drop me, I want you to drop me five, but I want to be able to do it on my own time at my own speed. You know, if I don't feel like having a drop in a month, then so be it.' I says, 'Maybe in two weeks I will take two drops, you know.' So, it was ... you know, I really had to get reassured from them, because they did some ... you know, they were fooling around with our lives so badly, at that point, well you couldn't trust them. They talk about trust, you know. It turned out that I was going along fine ... I knew what five felt like. When I dropped five, you know, I knew what it felt like. And I was working, so I knew a lot of the times ... when I was looking at the clock at three o'clock, wanting to get my methadone, that was odd for me.

So, I knew something was wrong. So, I says, 'You didn't drop me five,' I say, 'You dropped me ten, that is what it feels like.' She says, 'No, no, we didn't.' She says, 'Well, I will check.' She comes back and says that they did by mistake drop me to ten. You know, I still don't know whether to believe anything they said at that point. It was like that they were still fooling around with me. Here I am taking my own withdrawal. I am coming off, what more did they want? You know, they had to fool around with that, they couldn't leave well enough alone. [Evelyn]

The women interviewed claimed that their subjective experience of their own withdrawal was ignored by doctors and drug workers. Rather than respecting their requests, drug workers and doctors were perceived as playing games with the women when they were vulnerable and in need of support.

Another problem for long-term methadone patients was the unavailability of detox centres that would help them withdraw from other drugs. Some of the women on methadone were taking Valium, and, though they wished to withdraw, there appeared to be no options available to them:

Like I tried to get into detox because of Valium. I was on Valium and I tried to get off Valium. There was not one place that would take me, because I was on methadone. I could not go and get off the Valium, but stay on my methadone program. Not one place. [Evelyn]

Like the women on methadone studied by Rosenbaum and Murphy (1987), the women on methadone in this study faced many health- and drug-related problems that are not being dealt with effectively within current drug programs.

Ceasing Drug Use

Research suggests that many people are able to cease using drugs without the aid of drug treatment services (Alexander, 1990; Biernaki, 1986; Blackwell, 1983; Erickson, Adlaf, Murray, & Smart, 1987; Matthews, 1995; Peele & Brodsky, 1991; Reinarman, 1979; Stevenson, Lingley, Trasov, & Stansfield, 1956; Waldorf, Reinarman, & Murphy, 1991; Winick, 1962). Many of the women interviewed had ceased their drug use prior to this study, and others had ceased drug use for long periods of time before beginning to use drugs again. As mentioned above, many were able to cease their illicit drug use without the aid of drug treatment programs. Some of the women interviewed stated that they continued to use illicit drugs and legal methadone because the drugs made them feel 'normal.' The term 'normal' was used to describe a feeling of belonging and comfortableness with oneself and one's surroundings. Some of the women noted that they had never felt normal prior to using drugs. Others wished to regain the state of normalcy that they had experienced prior to their drug use.

Similar to Alexander's (1990) adaptive model of drug use, several women described how the use of illicit drugs made them feel normal:

You know, and of course when you are young, you know. People notice different kids ... I was never happy. I couldn't understand how people could smile and make jokes. I mean, the world was going to blow up, there are people starving, there is ... and all of it would get to me every day. I would remember this all the time. The first time that I ever got relief ... any true relief, was when I started doing heroin. It was almost like it put that extra skin on me that most people have so that they can deal with the world. And laugh and have a good time and enjoy a beautiful day. I couldn't do that. I never could, without heroin and I don't know why, to this day. I don't know why. [Theresa]

I don't know, people assume you're high, but most people who use narcotics just feel normal when they use. For me, I didn't feel normal unless I was using. So my quest was normalcy, not the high. [Hope]

One woman attending full-time university described how she felt normal prior to using drugs:

I felt like, before I did drugs I felt like I was normal. Even though I had been drinking beer I felt really normal ... I felt that, yeah, that I could fit into some pattern. I didn't feel totally ostracized the way I did after I used drugs. That's what I meant by normal, in the sense of how I felt after I used drugs, in the sense there must be something terribly wrong with me because, you know, I did this. [Morgan]

Others tried to recapture that sense of normalcy after they ceased using drugs:

But what a nice dream to go back to being somewhat happy and normal again. [Pat]

I enjoy doing other things, you know. I used to say before, oh I wish I was normal, [laughter] you know, and, you know, now I am normal. And I enjoy it. And I made a point of wanting to be normal. [Sue]

As Weil and Rosen (1993) noted in their interviews with drug users, the pursuit of feeling 'normal' appears to be a defining factor both in continuing drug use and in ceasing drug use.

For some of the women, the lifestyle associated with illicit drug use became too wearing. One low-income woman noted:

Yeah, it is mostly the bizarre nature of the lifestyle, that I just ... I couldn't live with it any more. It was making me crazy. There is so much ugliness there, there is so much ugliness in yourself that's hard to deal with, and the shit that other people are doing. Just ... it is just too ugly to have to live with. I mean, it was getting to the point where it is was, fuck, either kill yourself or get up and do something else. Get a gun or get over it. Because there are no other choices here. So, I got over it. [Pat]

Other women ceased their drug use after experiencing traumatic events in their lives. Two women of colour describe the situations that led them to stop using illicit drugs:

I guess what finally happened, my mum had been diagnosed with cancer of the blood about a year before this. And I guess in a lot of ways I was in a lot of denial, I couldn't imagine living without my mom, or my child. And I tried really hard not to focus on those things and I was sitting in my apartment one night and my mom was in the hospital literally dying and my son was there. And I just couldn't put the drugs down, get out of the house to go to the hospital to see the mom. And that's when it really hit me that this was too big for me, way more than I could handle. So I phoned this person to get me out of the house and I went up to the hospital and I got there and I, and they said to me, mum's sleeping very peacefully, so maybe you could just let her sleep. And I was gonna leave, and I got downstairs, and just something said to me if you don't do something now, you're not going to make it. And I just went up to my mum's bed and poured my heart out to God and just pleaded, and I've never used since. It's been thirteen months. [Greta]

When I met someone that didn't judge me, that accepted me the way I was and treated me as a normal person then that's when my life started to change, you know. And from that point on, you know, I started believing that I could do it. And I was a very bad addict. I was the kind of person you thought would never leave the street. [Sue]

Another woman on social assistance stressed the need for 'sanctuary' once the decision to stop illicit drug use was reached:

I think one of the most important things is to have a secure place to live. Being on this street, it is really tough to maintain a home of your own and addiction. And ... I don't think you can do it unless you have sanctuary to start with. That's really important for it. [Pat]

Overall, the women spoke about a wide range of experiences that influenced their decisions to stop using illicit drugs. There was no one magic formula, but many of the women noted that their success was due to the fact that they had stopped using illicit drugs because they themselves wanted to. One young mother of two children stated:

I think the main, main thing that I can say is, like, you can't do it for other people ... I really don't think it is possible to do it for anybody but yourself, really. Like, not even your kids. [Mary]

The women noted that attempts to stop using illicit drugs for their children, their family, or their social workers were not always effective. Furthermore, treatment is limited when compulsory. One Native Indian woman stated:

To tell you the truth, I don't think that any kind of treatment works. It has to be your own will. [Cindy]

Women are sceptical of drug treatment, for they have been forced, pressured, and directed to drug treatment even when the program did not fit their needs and when abstinence was unrealistic.

Shifting Patterns of Use

Many of the women interviewed discussed their shifting patterns of illicit drug use. Many had successfully quit using illicit drugs for long periods of time before starting to use again. One professional woman stated:

So you know, then that's the fearful thing because I quit those years and started again. And then quit for years and started ... Then I'll find a reason, I'll find the strength to quit or whatever. And then after a while that reason maybe doesn't exist any more. Or I'll start using again slowly, just a little bit, just occasionally and all that ... it's just been a real seesaw back and forth. [Gloria]

Defining drug use according to Alexander's (1990) 'continuum of involvement' illuminates the wide range of patterns of drug use. These are rarely static, as many of the woman interviewed noted.

In addition to using illicit drugs on and off, many of the women noted that they had successfully stopped using illicit drugs, but continued to use licit drugs. One woman of European heritage explained:

I don't know if I'm ever going to completely stop taking drugs because I still smoke, although I've cut down cigarettes and I think I will quit smoking cigarettes ... I still occasionally drink a few beers, but not often, but, you know, if I go out. And I'll still take painkillers if I feel that I need them. So, I think what I've done, I think, well, I'm not gonna do something crazy to get a drug. Well, I'm not gonna do that. [Morgan]

This woman was intent on leaving the criminal lifestyle associated with illicit drug use. By using only licit drugs she limited her chances of arrest, incarceration, and possible separation from her children. However, limiting drug use to only licit drugs is not an option for everyone.

Some of the women interviewed expressed their wish to be drug free, though at the time of the interview they had not been able to achieve their goal. One self-employed woman on methadone described how she hid her sorrow by acting arrogant:

Yes, it hurts my feelings really bad. I am ashamed of myself. I am really, really hurt inside ... I can feel how arrogant that I am being about the whole thing. Because really I mask the fact that I am really upset about it. Because I would love to be drug free. [Judy]

Other women were not attempting to achieve abstinence or occasional use of drugs, for their addictive drug-use patterns were directly related to their desire to suppress deeper painful experiences. One low-income woman whose children have been permanently apprehended by the Ministry of Social Services stated:

I try to get all this shit out of my head. All my family problems. You know, I was raped when I was younger. Being numb. Get all the old tapes out of my head. As soon as I get my life in order, you know, some of it, you know, then I could get off the drugs and stay away from it, got clean. I have done it before on my own. Then I go back to it. I get depressed, I get depressed. I want to commit suicide ... You see, with me, I won't face reality because I don't want to face reality. I don't want to face reality. Reality sucks and it hurts too much. [Julie]

For some women, addictive drug use is one way of adapting to a 'dire situation,' as Alexander (1990) states in his adaptive model of negative addiction.

Alternatives to Current Drug Treatment

During the interviews, the women discussed alternatives to current drug treatment policies and offered suggestions for reform. One woman in her early fifties noted how societal expectations are so much higher for illicit drug users than for licit drug users:

The person tries to quit smoking or to quit drinking and they fail, what do they do? They run down to the corner store, pick up their cigarettes or to the corner liquor store and pick their booze up. Now, if you try to quit heroin and you fail, it's not a matter of going to the corner store. It's a matter of going back on the street, and inevitably jail or death. And each time you quit or you try to quit and you fail, you face this, and this is to me where methadone comes in.

It's not that people want to go on methadone, it's that they get to a point in their life, they say, I've tried to quit, I can't quit. I read some [statistics] a few weeks ago that 95 per cent of people that lose weight gain it back. Now, how much harder is it to quit heroin? Now, some people would say that's debatable [laughs], y'know, but why ... would they single out, they take the heroin addict ... he's supposed to be unstable, like uh, bottom level of society ... at the very bottom, and yet they have greater expectations ... society in general ... of this lowly heroin addict than they do of our most stable citizen. How many times have you seen people that quit ... that are productive in the community and yet they ... when I say they can't quit smoking, I don't care the reasons. They're still smoking. Y'know, they can't do it and yet society says, well, if the heroin addict can't quit use of heroin, tough. They're going to have to face the consequences, which is going on the street, y'know ... it's that black and white. Well, nothing in life is black or white. And I think they have to come to more real ... y'know, face up to reality, that most people don't quit. There are some that do, and it's wonderful. [Linda]

Drug-treatment programs in Canada have been unable to face up to the fact that abstinence is an unrealistic goal for some drug users. Rather than punishing illicit drug users, it would be more beneficial to recognize the limitations of our current drug policy.

Alexander (1990) notes that imprecise definitions and labels have led to misleading information about people who use drugs. Official drug policy has no language for different patterns of drug use outside of problematic drug use. Drug policy and drug treatment are based on an abstinence model, and not all drug users are able to benefit from this model. The women discussed the harm of current drug-treatment policies and how illicit drug users, rather than the method of treatment, were personally held responsible for failure:

It is all set up to make you feel like a failure, because when there is only one method of treatment, if you don't fit in there. Well, that is the reason that ... one of the reasons that you became addicted in the first place. It is not like you ever fit in anywhere. So, it ... just ties into the whole thing. [Linda]

But mostly I think we have to look at how the medical profession in treatment also perpetuates myths about addicts and contributes to the addicts' perception of themselves as bad, immature, unable to be responsible. I think people who use drugs are responsible. Do have control. Using a drug doesn't give you a licence to behave in negative ways. When people say, 'Oh I was drunk,' or 'That's because I was addicted,' I don't buy that. That was the person being a jerk; the drug is not responsible. But I think the structure of our treatment centres makes it impossible for drug users to be honest, the laws make you feel dishonest. The things you do to get the drug, because you have to deal with the black market. So you begin to feel that is you. So instead of this focus on treatment centres, I'd like to see some recognition of how these centres can harm people, how they have become an industry. If we wanted real change in how people use drugs we should change society. Why do people want to use a drug? Why is that preferable? [Hope]

The women emphasize the ways in which current policy perpetuates myths about people who use illicit drugs. Rather than one model of drug treatment, the women interviewed asserted, many different programs should be available:

I think there should be a variety of programs because people react, y'know, differently to different programs. [Cathy]

Back to treatment, I think that whatever works for a person, whatever it is they feel will work. If the AA model is for them, go with it. If they want to do it alone, let them. We assume people need treatment, but I don't think so. Most users do stop on their own, without a detox centre or treatment, or counselling. But treatment has to recognize that each person is an individual, there's no universal answer, or answers. [Hope]

Other women discussed how the whole concept of treatment needs to change. Rather than just treatment, support of all types should be available to women:

Well, I think there should always be, you know, places for people to go to who need help. Places people can go to and get help right away to get help, when they decide to get help, not, you know, two weeks from now. A place where people can go to talk to people, but I don't think it has to be that big of a deal as it is. I don't think that people should go into a place and have their stuff searched. Which happened to me many times when you go into detox, even an alcohol detox I think they do it, like search you. So I mean, maybe that's for financial reasons because they don't want people in there wasting their time. But is the real reason for doing that, because if somebody is in there claiming they want to help themselves. The individual who is getting the help is going to determine what is the best help for them. Nobody else is the expert. There are no experts. What I'm saying is that there isn't any experts. So if I go for help, maybe need help financially, or maybe I need a place to sleep, someone [to] help me with my children. The rest of the stuff ... discussion maybe, and some new knowledge, but when you want it. [Morgan]

The women discussed the need to establish drug-treatment programs where infants could remain with their mothers. One women who had lost custody of three of her children to the Ministry of Social Services suggested that a supervised setting could be provided for mothers and infants labelled by the ministry as 'at risk,' rather than separating the infant from the mother:

A place to have some kind of drug rehab where they would put the babies and mothers together in a supervised setting. The baby wouldn't be at risk because they'd be supervised all the time. I think that would really help. It would help a lot more people than what we have now, which is nothing. [Liz]

Finally, the women interviewed discussed the need to broaden drug treatment to include maintenance programs, with other drugs available, and to stop penalizing drug users in maintenance who supplement their maintenance drug, especially under the current system. One professional woman on methadone noted how important it was to reduce harm rather than punishing drug users:

So, I think that it is really important for them to open that up ... there should not be just methadone either. They should have other forms of treatment. I mean if they take heroin or morphine ... you know, it should be other ways. So, what if people ... it doesn't really matter if they supplement. They might supplement for a while and still do other drugs on the side. But, there will be a time when that life just won't hold the same draw for them that it used to. For some it may be in their late twenties. Others it might be in their thirties. But, there will not be the human loss and the human misery and this revolving door, jail and losing babies and child welfare and addiction, that we have now. I mean, what have we got to lose? It's not working the way it is. So why can't they just try something different? [Carol]

Heroin maintenance

High on the list of methadone treatment reform, and drug treatment reform in general, was the need for heroin maintenance programs. All of the women who had been on methadone (36 per cent) stated that they would prefer to have legal heroin maintenance rather than the current policy of exclusive methadone maintenance programs.

I would rather have heroin. Because I think in the long run, I think that the heroin itself ... it is not as bad for you as methadone ... they are starting to know more about methadone, because they didn't at the time. Methadone gets right into your very bones and what not. You know, it gets ... it is such a horrible thing to come off of. Heroin is nothing to come off of. [Evelyn]

I mean if you were addicted to heroin, basically it is not to switch from one drug to the other. I mean that is not the answer either. I mean, if it was heroin that you had a problem with, well, then I think it should have been dealt on that basis, with heroin. You know, I think it would be much easier and I think that in the long run, my life would have been different, if I had ... either come off or stayed with the heroin, either on a treatment basis, exactly how a treatment program would go about ... I don't know, but I think basically, it should have just been, be there and we should be able to obtain it. I think health wise. A lot of people, things methadone does, heroin does not do to you. I know a lot of people have a hard time thinking that way. You know, heroin, oh my gosh!! You know, heroin is not a bad drug, you know, bad as far as side effects ... methadone has a lot of side effects ... you wouldn't have such a fear of coming off it. I mean methadone, you have that fear, you know. You know, you do something wrong, you go to jail, you are not going to get your methadone, I mean, the fear is always there of not being able to get your methadone one day. One day would make a difference ... So when you are always, in fear of that. Heroin is much easier to come off of. So, I think that people would have attempted to come off of heroin a lot better and more often. And if it took a couple of times, fine. You know, but if they were trying, they were trying. [Evelyn]

Because methadone is more difficult to withdraw from than heroin, many of the women discussed their fear that they might be subject to methadone withdrawal due to arrest and subsequent policy changes. The perceived health risks associated with methadone maintenance have continually been an obstacle for illicit drug users (see Rosenbaum & Murphy, 1987).

One woman discussed the official rationale for continuing methadone maintenance to the exclusion of other drugs:

The argument for methadone is so lame. That it is easier to dispense, longer acting. Why can't I have heroin cigarettes or opium? Why would they be difficult to dispense? They give methadone because it is the least desirable narcotic ... They are so worried that someone might actually like their drug, and drug treatment is not about liking what you're given. So methadone fits the bill, a mundane, heavy drug, unlike heroin. [Morgan]

Conclusion

Although some women are able to benefit from drug treatment, a majority of the women interviewed have been subjected to inhumane and cruel treatment. The separation of mothers from their children during drug treatment is a primary injustice. The prejudice many of the women experienced from social workers after admittance to drug treatment was also a deterrent to receiving what little help is available to mothers who use illicit drugs.

All of the women interviewed rejected the criminal model of addiction. Most also rejected the disease model, which requires total abstinence. Given the current system of criminalization, the women supported a medical model of addiction, though many expressed the need to move away from this model as well. They discussed a wide range of drug policy and drug treatment options that would incorporate a harm-reduction model and acceptance of drug users and drug use. They also discussed how decriminalization and legalization of drugs might allow the drug user to monitor drug use without the aid of 'experts.'

Methadone maintenance in Western Canada was also discussed. The women described the humiliating practices of supervised urine testing, body searches, and rigid policy that rendered methadone maintenance programs a failure for both the drug user and society. Reform of current methadone maintenance policies was suggested, with an emphasis on methadone patients on policy-setting boards, including government boards that direct policy. The inclusion of legal heroin in maintenance programs was advocated by all of the women who had been on methadone programs. The availability of other forms of drugs, such as heroin cigarettes and liquid opium, was also advocated.

In preference to drug treatment based on the disease model and the twelve-steps approach, the women claimed that treatment must be flexible, building on the drug user's perceptions and needs. Research that demonstrates that drug users can control their drug use and stop of their own volition suggests that the disease model and compulsory treatment are ineffective and harmful.

6

The Effects of the Criminalization of 'Narcotics'

It is evident that both Canadian and U.S. drug legislation were originally fuelled by moralism, racism, and economic concerns (see Boyd, 1984; Green, 1986; Musto, 1987; Solomon & Green, 1988). The Chinese in Western Canada and the United States, were perceived as an economic threat to white labourers after the completion of the railroads. In British Columbia, racism and economic fears directed at Chinese labourers culminated in a labour demonstration and riot in 1907. Mackenzie King, then the deputy minister of Labour, came to Vancouver to settle damage claims from the riots after being approached by two opium merchants seeking restitution (Boyd, 1984). King was surprised by the unregulated Chinese opium industry in Vancouver. However, it was not until several affluent Chinese Canadians complained about the opium industry that King saw a way of getting 'some good out of this riot' (Boyd, 1984, p. 115). King recommended that the importation, sale, and manufacturing of opium be regulated. Drug legislation was subsequently proposed, even though there was no pharmacological evidence to support drug prohibition (Boyd, 1984; Green, 1986; Solomon & Green, 1988).

Early advocates of drug prohibition in the United States were concerned that black Southerners be made to stop using cocaine (Musto, 1987), and that the Chinese in the West be made to stop using opiate derivatives (Morgan, 1978; Musto, 1987). Musto (1987) correlates the fear of Southern blacks who used cocaine with the high levels of lynching, and legal segregation, and voting laws that contributed to their political powerlessness. Although there is no evidence that black Southerners were participating in widespread cocaine use, racist fears culminated in the construction of punitive drug legislation that was intent on controlling a specific segment of the population – black Southerners. The public did not oppose early drug legislation and the broadening of police powers. They saw early drug legislation as controlling specific problematic segments of the population, which in Canada were the Chinese labourer and opium smoker (Solomon & Green, 1988) and in the United States were Southern blacks and western Chinese (Musto, 1987).

Solomon and Green (1988) state that there was an understanding that the original drug legislation in Canada would not be used against ordinary citizens. Middle-class Canadians were more likely to be addicted to patent medicines and products sold through the pharmaceutical industry than to opium. Drugs are most likely to be prohibited if they are associated with a disliked or powerless group (Beyerstein & Hadaway, 1990). By the 1920s, Chinese Canadians were portrayed in Parliament as spreading the disease of drug addiction throughout Canada (Solomon & Green, 1988). Stereotyping the drug user as 'other' has been a successful technique in promoting more punitive drug legislation. Race, class, and gender conflicts underlie North American drug legislation, and the aggressive social control of drug use has eroded the democratic structure of both Canada and the United States.

The 'war on drugs' mentality has contributed to the increased social control of drug users. Recently, the 'war on drugs' has become a 'war on women' (Bloom, Chesney-Lind, & Owen, 1994). Women who use illicit drugs are increasingly regulated and punished through legal sanctions and social service and medical policies (Clark, 1996; Gómez, 1994; Humphries, 1993; Humphries et al., 1992; Maher, 1992). Mothers who use illicit drugs are challenged on many fronts, for their behaviour is perceived as especially deviant by society in general, and in particular by the criminal justice system. Mothers who come into contact with the criminal justice system due to this bias are also vulnerable to race, class, and gender bias (Faith, 1993; Gómez, 1994; Griffiths & Verdun-Jones, 1989; Humphries et al., 1992; Martel, 1994; Paltrow, 1992; Rosenbaum, Murphy, Irwin, & Watson, 1990).

In addition, the artificially high illegal market prices of illicit drugs ensure that most poor users must occasionally engage in other criminal activities to support their families and their drug use. Mothers whose children are in the custody of the Ministry of Social Services or of relatives receive harsher sentencing than those whose children are in their care at the time of arrest and sentencing (Carlen, 1983; Daly, 1987; Eaton, 1985; Masson, 1992). Like medical and social services, the criminal justice system reinforces family values that are unattainable by most women in conflict with the law.

TABLE 6.1
Drug and Drug-Related Charges

Total Sample: 28	N	%
Total women with drug and drug-related charges	23	82
Incarceration under six months in past	21	75
Incarceration over six months in past	7	25

Drug and Drug-Related Charges

Twenty-four (86 per cent) of the women interviewed stated that Canadian narcotic laws have had negative effects on their lives. As well, twenty-three (82 per cent) of the women have been charged with drug, and drug-related, offences. The majority (75 per cent) of the women had spent short periods of time in jail upon arrest and sentencing for minor charges, and seven (25 per cent) had been sentenced to prison for longer periods, ranging from over six months to two and one half years (see table 6.1). Five (19 per cent) of the mothers interviewed lost custody of their children due to arrest and incarceration, and of those 19 per cent only one mother was able to regain custody of her child after her arrest.

Police activity, drug and drug-related charges, the fear of arrest for themselves and family members, and the stigma attached to arrest and prison time had left them sceptical about the legal system. Only four of the women interviewed claimed the law had not affected them, although three of them had been charged with drug offences, fraud, and prostitution:

I never really had any contact with the law, just when I was working downtown. I was never really in contact with the law. [Liz]

I don't think that I cared, really. I didn't think that I had much to lose. You know, I never thought of consequences, really. [Mary]

The Narcotic Control Act[1] has had many negative consequences, direct and indirect. Many of the women had accumulated several drug and drug-related charges since they had begun using illicit drugs. Often their charges were accumulated within a very short period of time:

Uhm ... trafficking heroin, trafficking cocaine, possession of stolen property. Many, many, many, many counts of prostitution, quite a few counts of possession, credit card ... and on and on and on. I have got a really, really big record that I put together in probably the space of four years. I have probably put together almost twenty charges. Yeah, once it starts ... it just goes from there. [Pat]

Well, I had forgery when I was, like, eighteen, ... I had a record, but I had never had a felony before, I had all misdemeanours. They were pretty small things. I had like a couple of ... like, in N.Y. I had ... loitering. Actually what I did last time, I didn't get busted for drugs, it was for writing cheques for money to get drugs. [Morgan]

Shoplifting, mini minors ... Oh, yes, possession of marijuana, but no narcotics charges. I have about six shoplifting and one possession of marijuana and that is all. [Judy]

Yeah, for drugs and alcohol. Yeah, altogether about ten convictions for about six, seven years. [Lori]

Arrest, drug charges, and convictions were primary effects of the law. However, drug-related crime is more a result of prohibition laws than of illicit drugs causing crime (Hadaway, Beyerstein, & Yondale, 1991). Johnson and Rodgers (1993) note that the high rate of arrest for minor charges demonstrates how the criminal justice system has failed women, for arrest and prison have failed to divert women from further criminal activity.

Many of the mothers, low-income and middle-class and professional women, spoke about how their lives were affected by the law in more indirect ways, including changes in their standard of living and their lack of legitimacy:

Well, directly the laws have taken a lot of ... a lot of loved ones away, in jail. Non-violent crimes, and we haven't hurt anybody. So, that directly affected my life. Indirectly, it makes you feel like you're not a real citizen of the country, because, you know, you don't feel legitimate, a legitimate person, because you are considered a criminal. And ... I think that when people are younger, they might almost be arrogant about it to cover up their hurt and shame. They can't be ... they are not real citizens, so they become sort of cocky and they hide behind [an] anti-establishment attitude. But I think that it does really hurt. Especially in your older years, when you do want to be ... you want your voice to be heard ... legitimate voice for your country. [Judy]

Well, yeah, I had to escape to the States. It threw my whole life off. I had almost a nervous breakdown by the end. I was stranded down there with two little kids. Their dad was in jail. Yes. It affected me. [Janet]

I feel like I have to have myself completely covered on all ... Because I don't really have any rights ... they are more or less privileges. [Morgan]

Oh God. Immeasurably. You know, in every which way possible. I don't imagine you want a long story on it? ... It depends on the year that you are talking about. I mean, drug laws have changed over the years and it has been given different inter-pretations ... okay, if you want my real honest opinion. If drugs had been legal, all drugs had been legal at the time that I finished high school ... I probably would be sitting in SFU or UBC right now as a professor. You know, an opium-smoking pro-fessor. I probably would have got my PhD ... to go to school is expensive and to be a drug addict is expensive. Unless you are a millionaire, you are not going to accomplish those two things. You are just not. [Theresa]

The women discussed their lack of credibility and voice in Canadian soci-ety and their vulnerability to persecution. Their status as illicit drug users had became a tool with which to silence them. For many of the older women, the recognition of their criminalized status was problematic, especially since they felt concerned about the political context of their lives, as illicit drug users. Hiding their illicit drug use from family, co-workers, and society in general added to their lack of legitimacy, and made it more difficult to feel that they would be able to participate in changing their social and political environment.

During the interviews, the majority of the women responded by draw-ing on their own experience with the law. Only 25 per cent of the women were in a stable full-time relationship at the time of the interviews. Two were widowed. However, some of the women spoke about the effects of the law in relation to themselves and their husbands:

I mean, I was married to my husband, who was an addict also. And, the four-teen years that I was with him, he did a lot of illegal things to support our hab-its ... So, in a way, he took a lot of the ... that kind of pressure off of me, but he ended up being in jail a great deal of the time. Then, during that period of time, I would be trying to supply him with drugs to keep going and to keep myself going ... A lot of it was a nightmare, basically. He ended up dying in jail with an overdose. He was really talented in all kinds of ways, but because of the laws, he ended up having ... to work doing illegal things to keep our habits going. And ... yes, it is just ... it didn't make it possible for either of us to do anything else with our lives. [Diane]

Oh, well, because of my husband, oh, definitely, yeah ... because P. went to jail for it. [Linda]

The lack of legitimacy, the loss of husbands and partners and family members, and the inability to create or sustain another way of life under the current drug legislation were evident in the women's responses. The artificially inflated prices of the black market and the amount of time and money required to sustain their illicit drug use left little time for other more conventional and creative pursuits. The death of loved ones was a constant backdrop during the interviews. As one women stated:

The cost is so amazing, so many people I knew growing up are dead now. You know, overdose, AIDS. It breaks my heart, because it didn't have to be that way. [Hope]

The violence generated by the 'war' on certain drugs affects not only individuals who use these drugs, but all members of society. Death is one horrific outcome of the war on drugs; others include police intervention and prison.

Fear of Arrest

As mentioned earlier, 44 per cent of the women interviewed stated that they were more concerned about the drug laws than about social service intervention (see table 6.2). Overwhelmingly, the women spoke about their fear of arrest and the consequences of arrest.

For the few women interviewed who had no criminal record, their sense of luck and fortune in not having been charged with a narcotic offence is evident:

Well, I've been fearful of being arrested. I have been involved in the criminal part of that, so I had cause to be very paranoid and nervous about it. I got through it without ever being arrested. I was really fortunate. [Greta]

No criminal record, but I'm telling you I believe in God, because there were a few times where I was ratted on. [Marg]

The rest of the women interviewed were not so fortunate. The threat of

TABLE 6.2
Level of Concern about Social Service Intervention and Drug Laws

Total Sample: 28	N	%
More concerned with drug laws than social service intervention	12	44
More concerned with social service intervention than drug laws	12	44
Drug laws and social service intervention equal concern	4	12

the law was often realized. The fear and destruction brought about via the law was apparent to both low-income and middle-class women:

I was so afraid of the cops. I was so afraid of being busted. [Pat]

I was more worried about the law [than about social services]. The consequences of arrest seemed much more severe. [Hope]

Because of their fear of arrest, many of the women were concerned about the quantities of illicit drugs they had carried in their personal possession, or had in their homes. Some stated that they only carried or dealt in small amounts because they did not want to be sentenced to prison:

But the only thing that I worried about ... I had a clean record, so, like, even if they catch me with a gram ... cause I would only ever have personal use on me. You're allowed to have so much if you're an addict ... and because it would be my first offence anyway, and I don't traffic, I didn't have to worry about getting charged with trafficking 'cause I wasn't doing it. [Karen]

Yes, because lucky enough I never ... I was always so frightened to go into jail, because I had a kid ... I never did anything big time. I was nothing but a gram dealer ... fortunately enough, I guess I had enough intelligence to know I couldn't get involved in anything big that would put me in jail. Suspended sentence was all I ever got. Thank god. Because that is ... I think that is really what saved me from ever going to jail. I knew that I just couldn't. [Because of the baby] ... and God knows what I would have done. Maybe I would have been a stool pigeon if it came to taking my kid away. All of those unthinkable things. The only option for me was a quarter per cent, 25 per cent is to get away with it. The rest of them are unthinkable, so I never did it. [Judy]

There was a lot of fear there. I think that is what ... why I didn't get into any trip too heavy, because I didn't want to go to jail. No way. [Sarah]

Many of the women were successful in maintaining a low profile and protecting their family life by dealing small quantities of illicit drugs. Other women who transported or sold larger quantities expressed their fear of arrest due to the fact that exporters and traffickers receive harsher sentencing, the maximum penalty being life imprisonment. One woman from a middle-class background stated:

I was a mule, I made lots and lots of money. Still, the worry, the stress, 'cause if you go down, you go down big. [Marg]

The women were aware that possession of large quantities of illicit drugs brought prison time. However, the chance to earn more money and to maintain a better standard of living for themselves and their children was appealing, especially when many of the women had no other monetary means outside of welfare assistance and drug dealing. Many of the white middle-class women had been dealing larger quantities of drugs than the rest of the women interviewed. For them, the narcotic laws presented a larger threat, based on their own experience of being charged with trafficking rather than simple possession. Furthermore, their association with partners who were dealing large quantities of illicit drugs and engaging in other more serious crime placed them at risk. Although these women had both economic and social resources that they could draw upon on arrest, the law was perceived as threatening.

Arrest and Prison

In 1994, women constituted about 14 per cent of all adults convicted under federal drug legislation in Canada (McKenzie, Williams, & Single, 1997, p. 293). In 1993, 5,631 adult women were charged with drug offences (including cannabis) (McKenzie et al., 1997, p. 318). In terms of pharmaceutical drug offences, women accounted for nearly a third of convictions, though they accounted for only 10 per cent of all cocaine charges (Health and Welfare Canada, 1991, p. x).

Like the Canadian cocaine users studied by Erickson, Adlaf, Murray, &

Smart (1987), the women in this study initially appeared to have little regard for drug laws. Some noted that they were fairly unconcerned about the law until they actually were faced with arrest and the consequences of arrest. This did not deter them from continuing their drug use; rather, their awareness of the law became an additional burden to bear in their already marginalized lives:

Well, the thing is, when I was at the most risk with the law was when I was least concerned about it because I was really, my concern was getting high. Well, not getting sick, not really staying high, not getting sick. And I put myself in extremely dangerous positions, with extremely dangerous people. And didn't, I mean I just blocked out stuff. When I got busted I had to face up to it. After that I did it again and I put myself in some really hazardous situations with people ... You are so detached from what real life is. [Gloria]

I think I was fairly cocky, and was fairly stoned and fairly arrogant at the time, so it wasn't a concern of mine until the first time I was arrested. I would have been, I don't remember, it was fourteen or fifteen. [Debbie]

To tell the truth, like, now, I really care about things, but before I didn't. I just didn't care at that time. [Cindy]

Other women had spent lengths of time in jail when they were juveniles. For some, their fellow inmates were friends and family. One Native woman stated:

I had no problems when I was in jail, actually, I actually did okay. It flew by. I knew everybody. They were all my street sisters. People I had worked with ... That's more why I never said anything to anybody [about being underage]. Because I had all these people here, that knew my family, knew my sister, or went out with my brothers. So I felt safe. [Jane]

Not all of the women had friends and family within the confines of prison. But all were introduced to criminal activity. Two young women noted:

I probably spent at least eight months or six-seven months in jail, in juvie jail, right? [Sue]

First offence and I got probation and then I breached my probation twice, so for two breaches of probation and one offence, I got six months. That's ridiculous ... a thirteen-year-old. I learned more in jail than I ever dreamed of knowing from the street. 'Cause you get ... that's where you get a mix of everybody. You don't get to pick who you hang out with. You're stuck in there with kids who've murdered. There was a Japanese girl in there for three years who was caught with all this heroin on her in the airport, who ended up getting killed after she got released ... I learned more from them. I mean, you hear about it, you want to try it. You get more curious ... [Karen]

For some women, their arrest and subsequent treatment within the criminal justice system encouraged, rather than diminished, further involvement with illicit drugs. One middle-class woman discussed her past drug conviction:

It was a bundle. Twenty-five caps. Which is nothing, but to them ... I just think of how ... I wasn't a criminal ... but, I mean, it put me on a path of no return and basically they said, at my trial and everything, you're a junkie. And I thought, you want to see a junkie, I'll give you a junkie. It was like self-fulfilling prophecy. I was just so devastated ... and bought into the whole stereotype, as I say, of what a junkie is. That I just thought, well, if that's what you think I am, then I might as well be that. [Carol]

Being sentenced to prison was also problematic when the women became adults. The stigma, long sentences, and loss of family were deeply felt. Some women described the reality of prison time and the restrictive and humiliating process of criminalization. Two women from working-class backgrounds noted:

I mean, being in jail, it totally strips you of any self-worth that you have. After people handle you, and you know, put chains on your ankles, and transport you to places with shackles on your feet ... with shackles on your feet, with your hands tied around your waist with a belt. And after you're treated that way, after a while you give up a part of yourself and I think that they take it from you. And you give it up because physically, you just don't know, mentally you don't know any better and physically you have to. And a lot of people never get it back and a lot of people, if you expect a certain behaviour ... then you will get that behaviour from them. And if you say that all drug addicts are the lowest things on earth, then that's what they'll be. And if you start treating all people with respect, then, you know, you start seeing improvement. But as long as we have this myth about drugs and about what it is. And we have people drinking alcohol, people who work in

these drug enforcement agencies that go home and drink booze and smoke cigarettes and then come out on the street the next day and bust somebody for crack
or heroin. It is a double standard. [Morgan]

I got two years less a day. And that was another problem I see with the laws and
the way the whole judicial system is set up. I think it would have been better for
me to go to the penitentiary, where I would have had more chance to attend university, 'cause I already had my Grade 12 finished ... The jail wasn't set up for
long-term people like ... the average length of stay there was about a month. And
I saw women come and go, like, four and five times, and that's really hard, to be in
jail and see ... people are preparing to go and then they are out and then they are
back ... And the tension in the jail, I mean, there was a few people that as soon as
they came in the whole jail was just, like, you were always watching your back and
they just terrorized everybody. [Carol]

Incarceration revealed the inadequacy of the penal system in relation
to women (Faith, 1993). Few services such as education and drug treatment were available to the women in this study. As well, the social fiction
dividing illicit and licit drugs was blatant. Shackling women and treating
them as if they were 'dangerous offenders' only exacerbated already distrustful relations between the women and the criminal justice system.
Incarceration was difficult for the women; separation, and loss of children while in prison was doubly traumatic for Native and non-Native, low-
income, middle-class, and professional mothers:

That meant that I was [to prison] for seventeen months. And when I got out, B.,
L.'s dad, had L. long enough that he thought, well, we will just get her out of my
life. I was an inconvenience to them then. They had done this whole thing of having the nice little nuclear family and they pretended that L. was their kid, between
him and his ... it was really his stepmother. And stepsisters. They basically changed
his name. They divorced me completely from his life. [Carol]

Well, it completely affected my life, for one thing I spent time in jail for drug-
related crimes ... They affected me a lot. With both my children, with my first
child ... that was when I had to go to jail, I was gone almost three years and we
were separated. And I had a lot of problems with my child due to the separation.
Because of the separation. And a lot of problems with myself. [Morgan]

I was arrested for possession of cocaine; the kids were apprehended. And I felt
really, really upset because I thought I'd lost them for good that time. [Cathy]

I didn't even care about the going to jail, although I thought that would be pretty hard. That was a little frightening ... it was the separation from the kids. [Janet]

Women who are sentenced to prison often lose custody of their children, for there are few prisons that allow children to reside with their mothers, and then only if their children are under two years of age (Faith, 1993). The majority of women who are sentenced to prison are mothers (Faith, 1993). Most of them are poor and single parents and the separation and loss of their children are of primary concern (Faith, 1993; Simpson, 1989). Women who have sole responsibility for their children feel the impact of prison more deeply than do men (Johnson & Rodgers, 1993). As noted earlier, women who have their children living with them at the time of arrest and sentencing are likely to receive a more lenient sentence than those who no longer have custody of their children (Carlen, 1983; Daly, 1987; Eaton, 1985; Masson, 1992).

The criminal justice system serves to reinforce family values, and the loss of custody leads to subsequent harsher penalties. There appears to be no recognition of the extended family, and this has negative implications, especially for Native Indian women in Canada. For these women, children may be raised by a member of the family, rather than by the birth mother (Monture, 1989). Twenty per cent of the children born to the mothers interviewed were in the care of relatives. The decision to place a child in the care of other family members was judged by the criminal justice system as a sign of neglect and poor mothering. But for the birth mothers the decision to have other family members raise their children was an act of good parenting. In the case of one woman of European heritage whose drug use was escalating, her middle-class family offered a safe and familiar environment for her children, rather than a life fraught with unpredictability and possible child apprehension:

I didn't want to do that to my kids, so I went to my family ... [and said], 'The only thing that you can do for me is to keep my kids safe.' [Pat]

Other children were raised in an extended-family situation, and their mothers' drug use was irrelevant to this arrangement.

Police Surveillance

Because of their visibility as illicit drug users, many of the women were in contact with the police, either on the street, during drug arrests, or in their homes. The criminalization of drugs and the resulting illegal market have created a situation in Canada of increasing criminalization of individuals. Illicit drug use is considered a 'victimless' crime, and it is difficult for law enforcers to know who is actually using, buying, and selling drugs. Most illicit drug users do not complain to the police, nor are they easily identifiable by other people in the general population. Accordingly, the police have developed many proactive and controversial procedures to obtain narcotic arrests and convictions (Alexander, 1990; Cohen, 1985; Solomon, 1988; Stoddart, 1982; Wisotsky, 1986).

Informants, disguised police officers and undercover agents have been frequently employed since the criminalization of narcotics. Stoddart (1982) explores the lifestyle of undercover agents, noting their disregard of the law and their abuse of the people they are interacting with. The police routinely trick and force people into selling drugs in order to arrest them. Undercover agents break the law, use and sell narcotics, violate trust, and encourage criminal activity in order to arrest illicit drug users. These practices are dangerous, in the sense that society sanctions police criminality in order to persecute illicit drug users (Alexander, 1990; Cohen, 1985; Solomon, 1988; Stoddart, 1982; Wisotsky, 1986).

All of the women interviewed spoke about their problematic relationships with the police, the law, and society in general. For the majority of the women, their visibility as illicit drug users in Canada led to police persecution:

I remember years ago, in the early 70s, we used to call the streets the front lines because that is where the war was really taking place at that time. [Theresa]

It's not a war on drugs, it's a war on people. [Linda]

It really is a 'you and them' situation when you are using. And they play that to the hilt, too. I think they are just as into this game of cops and robbers, sort of a glorified image of themselves, but really that's all self-created, there's no reason to have this cops-and-robbers attitude around drugs. I just can't see police, RCMP, giving this position up, because how could they justify their existence for all those years? And where else could they get to play that game, with narcs, and undercover agents, and wire tapping? [Hope]

Alexander states that the war on drugs in Canada fits the 'pattern of a war of persecution' typified by the way in which heretics were historically treated (1990, p. 50). The warlike activities associated with the criminalization of drugs in Canada has subjected an increasingly large segment of the population to government-sponsored surveillance and violence. In addition, women who do not fit the familial model of good wife and mother are less protected by police (Edwards, 1987; Radford, 1987). The women interviewed described how the police were conditioned to respond to them cruelly, as if they were not human and had no human rights.

Well, they have to be trained, you know ... we've all met police who're civil, who can talk to you. But on the other hand, ... I don't know how many years ago ... we got a guard dog and it was trained. The dog was a year old. Gentle. This dog was as gentle ... on command she was grabbing hold of here. And that's what the drug squad used to remind me of. I thought, how can they be walking along ... a dog ... how can they, on command ... they become like ... the dog would run and grab you ... I don't know whether it's vicious. Now here you have ... here's a man sitting in a park, gets out of a car, and within seconds ... I couldn't do that. I couldn't get that hate, that anger, within ... you know, if somebody came up and attacked my family I could, I know I could, I could kill somebody if somebody attacked my family. But to sit in the car, or just wherever and then within seconds ... how do you get worked up to that, where you can kick a door down and choke someone? [Linda]

And for cops, they can be real problems. I mean they can want anything, money or sex. For just pure harassment of you. [Theresa]

They were also very cruel, treated you very badly the police. And really condescending. You know? They couldn't find any visible marks of using, so they would say crude remarks. 'So where do you fix? In your snatch?' [Sarah]

When I was still hooking ... and was using drugs or selling drugs of course the cops were always, always a concern to you. Uhm ... but it wasn't because of anyone finding out any more. It was just because of the mess they were gonna make of the place and who was going to have to get kick[ed] around and, you know, shit like that. So, I don't think that anybody scared me after a while. [Theresa]

The 'threat' of illicit drugs is perceived to be so great that government and police intervention is viewed as 'noble' rather than suspect (Hadaway et al., 1991). Consequently, much of Canadian society believes it must be protected from illicit drug users. One middle-class woman discussed how the police treated her depending on the type of drug involved:

So, heroin addicts, you bust them and you treat them a certain way. And if some-body is getting busted for marijuana, you treat them like it is not a big deal ... But you get treated differently, depending on the drug. I don't know if that is neces-sary. [Sarah]

Although heroin, marijuana, and cocaine were subject to the same penal-ties under the Narcotic Control Act, police may demonstrate discretion when choosing whom to arrest on drug charges. And Canadian judges have demonstrated discretion through sentencing. Heroin offences receive the harshest penalties. Marijuana offences receive the most lenient penalties (Health and Welfare Canada, 1991).

Even after some of the women had ceased using illicit drugs and engag-ing in other criminal activity, the police continued to contact them. Once they had been identified as illicit drug users, the women found it difficult to achieve another status in the eyes of law enforcers, regardless of their cessation of illicit drugs. Some of the women noted that when the police were actively pursuing their male partners, they were harassed and often set up:

When I was with T.'s dad and we would get busted, they would ... those laws affected me in that they used me to get him ... Well, they just busted me and all of my family, to wheel and deal. So that they could get what they wanted. [Sarah]

I had cops fuck with me so bad. You know, especially if you are in a drug-dealing relationship with a man. They always fuck with the woman on little itty bitty shit though. For they'll keep harassing her on ... I mean I have had tickets for crossing on the wrong side of the crosswalk, for spitting, for dropping a cigarette butt, for a napkin flying out of a bag, any reason to give a ticket or harass you or get [you] into the paddy wagon ... I mean, you know. Thirty days' time for a joint. For ... having your name on the lease. I am charging you with all of the stolen property. Even if they know it is not yours. Anything ... you know a lot of that is because usu-ally the guy in the relationship is the one buying some drugs on a larger scale and so ... they think the woman is the security in the relationship. So they always try to yank her out first. Not to do her any good though. Just as a jolt. [Pat]

We were constantly hassled in this small town ... They never found anything because he really did stop dealing when we moved in together, but the cops just wouldn't let him be. Actually, it was the RCMP. [Hope]

Their visibility as illicit drug users led to harassment even when the woman had no criminal record and had ceased using illicit drugs. One woman who has been on methadone maintenance for many years described how the police continued to harass her because of their suspicions about past drug dealing:

I have no criminal record ... They don't come to the door any more but we are still harassed. Always, always, always. [Marg]

Some women were able to avoid police harassment when they were able to maintain a conventional lifestyle, did not live in poverty, and had not acquired a criminal record. Two women noted how differently they perceived the police now that they lived a more conventional lifestyle and had ceased illicit drug use:

Like, I used to hate the police, used to hate them. Now, it is, like, I don't know, it has changed. I don't know how and when and all, but I just changed. [Cindy]

I'm so straight now. And you see, my charges were dropped. So I don't have that ... I don't even have a dislike of the law now. Now I actually look at them ... myself, from where I'm sitting, I look at them with pleasant eyes, that they're here to protect me again. I mean, I've done a hundred-and- eighty-degree shift. Or three-hundred-and-sixty-degree shift because I'm not illegal at all. So I like them protecting us. But it's a whole new way of looking at it. I don't think of them as pigs any more. 'Cause I'm not on the other side. I don't do anything illegal. [Janet]

For some women who did not bear the stigma of a criminal record, and who were able to re-enter conventional society, the police no longer were perceived as the enemy. However, as one young woman stated:

Like, I'm glad the police ... if there was no cops I wouldn't want to be around. But they definitely need to, educate a little more, especially with the police working downtown. They need to educate them ... from a different point of view, from a different ... Not from a legal, necessarily a legal standpoint, because it's the way that they act. If they start off and they come on strong and get in your face ... everyone downtown reacts. Anybody down there will react. And if you act a little different and try to show them respect, it doesn't mean you're kissing their ass. Then they'll react with a little more respect back to you, whether you're a cop or not. If you deal with them as a human, not as a 'drunken fucking Indian' or 'spic' or 'god damm junkie.' [Karen]

Another woman in her late forties described her sense of security now that she no longer participated in illegal activity; however, this sense was partially derived from no longer being witness and victim to the power that the police wield when persecuting illicit drug users:

Yes. It feels really, really good now. Like, I guess it is just the power that the police and the system have. [Sarah]

The Controlled Drugs and Substance Act gives licence to police practices that most Canadians would find horrifying in another context. Most women do not choose to live outside the law; rather, many women have limited choices and act within the confines of economic, social, and political constraints.

Drug Dealing

The artificially high prices of illicit drugs make it difficult for many women to finance their illicit drug use through legitimate means, especially if they are poor. Until recently there has been little information available about women who sell drugs. However, recent studies have contributed to and challenged past perceptions (see Dunlap, Johnson, & Maher, 1997; Maher, 1995; Morgan & Joe, 1997). As Waldorf, Reinarman, & Murphy (1991) highlight in their study of cocaine users, the image presented by the media of the ruthless drug dealer is faulty. In fact, most drug dealers 'drift' into dealing. To build on David Matza's sociological premise, drug dealers are neither 'compelled nor committed': 'Users often sell to defray the costs of their own supplies, to get better quality drugs, or to assist friends and associates in buying higher quality drugs at quantity prices' (Waldorf et al., 1991, p. 76).

Many women participate in drug dealing to finance their family responsibilities and illicit drug use (Dunlap et al., 1997; Morgan & Joe, 1997; Maher, 1995; Rosenbaum, 1981; Taylor, 1993). Rarely do women set out to 'deal drugs.' Rather, the combination of their economic situation and their illicit drug use facilitates a 'drifting into dealing.' This drift may only entail pooling money with other friends to obtain a better deal, or selling small quantities to support their own drug habits. A small minority of women drug users sell larger quantities (Dunlap & Johnson, 1996; Morgan & Joe, 1997). Traditionally, women have not been integrated into the larger 'cartel' type of drug dealing that is so avidly popularized by the media. Women are sometimes offered the role of the 'mule' – smuggling

TABLE 6.3
Participation in Illegal Activities

Total Sample: 28	N	%
Selling drugs and transporting drugs	14	54
Prostitution	11	39
Other	3	11

and transporting illicit drugs – but this type of activity is less lucrative. Nevertheless, it carries severe legal penalties, including life imprisonment.

Recently, Morgan and Joe (1997) examined the use and selling of methamphetamine in the United States. They note that, for women, the option of selling methamphetamine was often 'the best opportunity to successfully achieve a level of independence and control over their life' (Morgan & Joe, 1997, p. 99). For many women, selling drugs brings security, independence and increased self-esteem (Dunlap et al., 1997; Morgan & Joe, 1997).

Eighty-nine per cent of the women interviewed partially or totally financed their drug use through illegitimate means at different times. Similar to Fields and Walters's (1985) findings related to legal activities and illicit drug use, over a third of the women partially financed their illicit drug use by legitimate means through full- or part-time work. Outside of legitimate means, drug dealing was the most prevalent financial choice for the women interviewed (see table 6.3), followed by forgery, prostitution, shoplifting, transporting of drugs, and B & Es (break-and-enter). Selling the drugs appeared to offer a means to finance one's drug use as well as to obtain economic security, even though this was rarely realized. Seventy-one per cent of the women interviewed were on welfare assistance at the time of the interview. Drug dealing offered a means to supplement an income that was insufficient. Like cocaine users and sellers in Waldorf et al.'s (1991) study, and the male drug dealers studied by Hagedorn (1994), the women interviewed maintained ties with conventional society and perceived their drug dealing as a means to supplement their income.

Over half of the women (54 per cent) had participated in dealing and transporting drugs. Many had participated in dealing only small amounts in order to finance their own drug use. Many supplemented their drug habits by visiting doctors in order to get legal prescriptions. Double-doctoring was common, especially prior to the practice of using triple prescriptions, a system that closely monitors the prescribing of specific legal narcotics by providing a copy of the prescription to Pharmacare doctors, and pharmacists, in order to control use. Eleven per cent of the women obtained their drugs through legitimate means, and other activities. Thirty-nine per cent of the women had worked as prostitutes, although 14 per cent of these had also dealt drugs. Participation in criminal activity fluctuated according to need and availability. Many of the women (36 per cent) participated in methadone programs either for short periods (up to three months) or for longer periods (up to twenty years). During that time, they stated, they ceased or limited their illegal activities. In addition, having a partner sentenced to prison might mean that the woman had to find other means to support her habit. Alternatively, price increases on the illegal market might necessitate visiting doctors for prescription drugs.

In short, one's social and economic situation most often predicted what type of activity one might engage in to finance illicit drug use, as well as one's own beliefs about certain activities. For example, two of the women stated that they were not able to participate in prostitution when they were poor, not because they thought it was morally wrong, but for other reasons:

Well, I just felt so corny, actually. I couldn't ... I didn't think, yes, I don't think that I felt sexy enough to stomp around like that. [Mary]

I remember being so broke, and really wanting to work the street. But you know what stopped me? Not my concern about whether it was right or wrong. No, I couldn't get myself to try because I was afraid that no john would actually want to pay money to be with me. What a fool I was. My self-esteem was so low, I couldn't imagine it. Little did I know it has nothing to do with being attractive anyway. But looking back, I guess it's okay it worked out that way, because I didn't need more things in my background to be stigmatized about. I have enough without prostitution too. [Hope]

The majority of the women interviewed had few choices in relation to financing their illicit drug use. For the poor women interviewed who were dependent or addicted to illicit drugs, artificially inflated black market prices generally ensured that a conventional lifestyle would be impossible to obtain, let alone maintain. Some women supplemented their incomes through prostitution, although this choice often led to increased visibility as illicit drug users, and to lengthy criminal records.

Prostitution

Researchers have written about the link between prostitution and illicit drug use (Goldstein, 1979; Inciardi, Lockwood, & Pottieger, 1993). Some women who use illicit drugs engage in prostitution to finance their income. However, Morgan and Joe (1997) challenge this direct link in their research on methamphetamine users in the United States. The low rate of prostitution in Morgan and Joe's (1997) and Taylor's (1993) studies of female drug users is consistent with this study, where fewer than half (39 per cent) of the women interviewed had worked as prostitutes. Moreover, drug use did not always precede prostitution. Rather, poverty initiated an interest in prostitution (Rosenbaum, 1981). However, Lowman and Fraser note that drug use most often increases after women begin to work as street prostitutes (1995, p. 62). All of the women had worked as street prostitutes, though statistically street prostitutes represent 'a small portion of the market.' Street prostitution exposes women to more danger than does working in more protected environments, such as massage parlours or escort services (Shaver, 1993, p. 157). Researchers note that many street prostitutes survived physical and sexual abuse in their youth (Lowman & Fraser, 1995). The street offered only an illusion of refuge, for women were subject to further violence and police harassment there (Johnson & Rodgers, 1993; Lowman, 1991; Lowman & Fraser, 1995). Many women enter street prostitution as juveniles (Lowman, 1991). However, the majority of street prostitutes in Vancouver work independently of pimps (Shaver, 1993). Some of the low-income women described their first experiences working as juvenile prostitutes:

And then the first time I had to go out, I had to work the street, you know. When someone picked me up I just cried. I cried to this guy, you know. He stunk, and he was disgusting. He was fat and ugly, and, you know, and I looked very, very young when I was that age and ... I cried, you know. I didn't do anything with the guy, but I cried to him. You know, I said, 'Listen, my boyfriend is going to beat me up and ... get really mad at me if I don't bring in any money.' And then he got mad at me too. And he goes, 'Well [why] do you think I should give you the money ... You didn't do anything.' And then finally I was crying so hard and everything he just gave me twenty bucks and said, 'Here. Get out of the car right here' ... My boyfriend at the time, he was watching, you know. Well, he was ... off in the bushes to make sure nothing happened to me. So I got out of the car and he saw every-thing happen and he said, 'Well that's the way to do it.' [Sue]

Street prostitutes are often the victims of violence. One young woman describes being attacked by a john:

One problem with the industrial areas is if they start to attack you there's no house to run to. But I found once, when I was being attacked and I ran around, and I knocked, they wouldn't let me in. It was just like in the movies ... they wouldn't answer the door ... He drove me all the way ... I think it was North Van. North Van. And he wouldn't let me out of the car. I was trying to hit telephone poles, cops didn't stop ... people didn't stop ... I'm yelling and screaming. I finally get out of the car, he's chasing me with the car as I'm running, and people would not answer their doors. I said, 'Can you just call the cops, you don't have to let me in ... call the cops. I'm not gonna' ... but I can see their point, too. You know, you see some ... you know, I can see their point of view, too. But ... to think that what if I was just jogging, because I didn't look like a hooker then. I could have just been anybody. [Karen]

Prostitutes are much less able to exercise their rights than other women and are subject to considerably more violence (Edwards, 1987; Lowman & Fraser, 1995; Radford, 1987).

The women also spoke about their interaction with undercover police, for the use of surveillance and undercover police activity is common prac-tice in regulating prostitution as well as narcotic offences. One young African-American woman noted:

No, I didn't get caught for drugs. I ended up getting caught for prostitution ... Which was really sad because I never actually ever slept with anybody for money. I tried to do it twice and both times ... the first two people that I talked to were cops ... It took five years for me to try again after the first time. Then I tried again and it happened exactly the same way ... I just say, well, obviously, I was not meant to be a hooker, right? I fought for one [charge], actually. It was entrapment, the guy asked me like six times and I said no, no, no, no, no. Yeah, then he told me that I could have one hundred bucks. So I said okay, well ... I told him to go away ... He said, 'God, no one has ever said no to me before.' He was getting all sort of offended, even. You know, it was like, well, God ... I said, 'No, like, look.' But finally when he told me how much money he had. 'Well, how far did you say that you had to go?' And ... I don't know, we walked down there and, well, you are under arrest. Oh, no, I had a feeling all of a sudden. It was strange, though. You know, how you get that feeling just before, that they know everything. It is always too late ... I knew ... all of a sudden, I knew he was going to pull out a badge instead of a key. And I sort of waited to see, like I could have just said, 'Oh, on second thought, no, I'm lying' and left. But, no, I just had to wait and see if it was true ... But what pissed me off was how many times he asked me ... When I was getting fingerprinted, because I didn't show up at court. I had missed court and he put me up for failing to appear and his partner was the one that fingerprinted me. And I was describing the way that I got caught. He said, 'I remember you.' That sounds like something my partner would do, he said. I was, like oh God! [Mary]

Police subject women working as prostitutes to an array of under-handed practices in order to lay charges, just as undercover police entrap illicit drug users. Upon their arrest the stigma attached to prostitution greatly affects women. Sometimes they even plead guilty to charges that might have been dropped:

Yes, I just went and pled guilty, because I didn't want them talking about it, because I know too many people in those courtrooms. Oh, God. I knew, like, I could go through the whole trial thing and probably win, but I just couldn't be bothered. I didn't want to be spending time in court. I just didn't want it spread around. Like, the more it is time to go to court, The more times I am bound to see people that I know in there. [Mary]

I guess when I first started hooking out of poverty and I had the kids with me. I hadn't really got into any ... any drug abuse ... I started the prostituting first. It was a way to get out of my finance problems which were killing us. And ... I was so afraid of the cops. I was so afraid of being busted. I was ... I was afraid of anyone finding out what I was doing. It was like ... and I had no idea what the consequences were of what I was doing, but, mostly ... was I didn't want anybody to know. And having run ins with the law meant people finding out. [Pat]

Poverty, not drugs, is often the impetus to engage in prostitution, although illicit drug use is often an associated factor (Erickson & Watson, 1990; Johnson & Rodgers 1993; Lowman & Fraser, 1995; Shaver, 1993). For many women, especially for street prostitutes whose working conditions consist of long hours and dangerous streets, prostitution is not very lucrative. Working the streets once children are born often changes a woman's lifestyle as well. The responsibility of maintaining a family and a drug habit and working the street was common to 34 per cent of the women interviewed. All the women interviewed were low-income when they engaged in prostitution:

The second time A. was about two or three ... Two, two and a half. And again ... the dope was really bad on the streets and because my husband wasn't working and all this. I was screwed. You know, I hadn't worked for years. I am not exactly frightened ... you know, to keep up the family money going. You know, in that manner. So, I went back to work. And ... I guess having a child sort of changed this situation, that ... you know, there was a little more guilt, because again, I mean, you are working long hours out there to make money. That was a time that was in the early 80s, in the depression as well. I mean, I knew girls that stood out there for ten hours some nights and made no money. You know, you would see them there at eight o'clock the next morning, you know. You just want to cry for them. [Theresa]

It is probably important to know that I have been hooking for a while. That is how I got to doing cocaine and things. You can't really look after kids all day and hook all night and back again. It got me out of my poverty problem, which was cool for a while, but keeping up the lie with everybody about what I was doing with my life. Everyone was pretty content to go ... well, at least she has some money now, you know, and the kids have bikes and clothes and this and that. [Pat]

As long as their prostitution was hidden, the mothers were perceived as taking care of their primary responsibilities. However, once their prostitution became public through arrest, the law did not protect them; the women became aware of the danger both johns and police presented to them, and often they became hardened to the subsequent police harassment they would experience:

Over the years ... when I was still hooking and ... and was using drugs or selling drugs of course the cops were always, always a concern to you. [Pat]

For a woman who lacked other marketable skills, if her drug habit increased or if drug dealing became less feasible, prostitution often became a solution to financial difficulties. In short, poverty led the women in this study to work as prostitutes. One woman lived with a drug dealer and, when their relationship ended, she began to engage in prostitution:

At first I just lived with a dealer, and whatever, and when the last one went to jail I was up so high, the amount was so high every day, it wasn't possible to do it that way. There wasn't enough money for everyday things. [Greta]

The difficult life of the street prostitute who is participating in heavy illicit drug use is captured in one woman's assessment of her life when she was poor and addicted to cocaine:

Women on the street are battered about between men and the law, back and forth, back and forth. Prostitutes' life is between a fuck and a fix. A fuck and a fix. [Pat]

For some women, prostitution and illicit drug use often went hand in hand. The double stigma of illicit drug use and prostitution was evident as the woman's criminal record expanded. One Native Indian woman described her early criminal record:

Prostitution. Prostitution, failure to appear, breach. [Sue]

Unlike her male counterpart, the female drug user is often more visible to police scrutiny when she engages in prostitution (Lowman, 1991). Within a short period of time she can acquire a lengthy criminal record that often has far-reaching effects in terms of sentencing and of her ability to keep her family intact. As previously mentioned, women who engage in prostitution are more likely than their male customers to receive criminal records and punitive sentencing (Shaver, 1993).

Race, Class, and Gender

The race, class, and gender issues underlying drug legislation and enforcement have been explored by critical researchers (Alexander, 1990; Blackwell, 1983; Boyd, 1983, 1984, 1990; Brecher & The Editors of *Consumer Reports*, 1972; Faith, 1993; Gómez, 1994; Humphries et al., 1992; Maher, 1992; Preble & Casey, 1969; Reinarman, 1979; Rosenbaum et al., 1990; Szasz, 1974). Poor women and women of colour are most vulnerable to police harassment and arrest (Adelberg & Currie, 1993; Bloom et al., 1994; Chunn & Gavigan, 1991; Faith, 1993; Johnson & Rodgers, 1993). The unequal treatment in police discretion and later in sentencing was evident to the women interviewed.

Native women who were interviewed acknowledged the existence of institutionalized racism within the judicial system. Some believed that they could respond to it proactively:

If you stand up for yourself and you don't cower in a corner like you see some people do. If you stand up for yourself, then they know that you are not a weak person ... so just because I am Native, that is not going to stop me from saying what I want to say. [Cindy]

Standing up for themselves empowers women by giving them a sense of agency. Unfortunately, current drug legislation and race and class bias undermine personal attempts to maintain agency. Research that demonstrates that criminalized women, and women who use illicit drugs, suffer from poor self-esteem is simplistic. As Gavigan notes, poor self-esteem may be a result of 'being labelled and incarcerated' (1993, p. 228). Racism is also problematic; Monture-Okanee, Thornhill, and Williams (1993) describe how racism is a type of violence that can't be touched or seen, which renders it invisible.

For women who are arrested, the racial and class composition of prison is a lesson in Canadian judicial inequality. One woman of European heritage described her time in prison:

And the loss, like, it just floors me, like the whole thing about the Native population ... It was, like, 87 per cent Native women. In for stupid little things, like ... I mean the average stay was a month. I mean where were their children? Their children were either taken away or in bad situations. [Carol]

And a Native Indian woman noted:

I never felt like I belonged, being called a dirty Indian, or this or that. [Cathy]

One young woman of European heritage spoke about her perception of racism and police activity in downtown Vancouver:

They ... how to explain it ... it's not so much that they don't hassle white people, but Natives and Spanish they definitely hassle more. They definitely, because it's the stereotype. With Spanish, they're all drug dealers ... but that's downtown. Right, some of them aren't and it's not fair to the ones that aren't. But they do get hassled more. Natives get hassled more ... But it's almost like they're prejudiced not because they're personally prejudiced but because the policy ... it's just because of patterns that happen downtown. That they're just going with the patterns and it's not really that they're personally prejudiced. Some of them are. But, yeah, I definitely got hassled less but that's also because of the way I appeared, too. I mean, there's a lot of white girls that dressed like tramps that got hassled, too. I just tried to keep as low-key and kind of plain and not draw attention to myself and keep quiet and low-profile. [Karen]

Another woman of European heritage described her interaction with the police from the vantage point of class and her status as a single mother while living in a housing project:

Well ... they are all negative. I mean you always ... you are given a negative reaction right away from everybody. I mean you have ... the police come for an unrelated incident ... they are coming in to a housing project, I am on welfare. I am a single mother with a teenage daughter. Even without the knowledge of anything else. It is like, 'XXX,' right away. [Evelyn]

In addition, the women spoke about their difficulty in protecting themselves when charged with a criminal offence due to their low economic status:

My family was working class, poor, but then I was on welfare too and a single parent. Life is so different now that I have moved from that class. I am treated so differently. I'm glad that I had a chance to see how white, middle-class people are treated, because that is a new experience to me. Being raised working class and then on welfare, no education, no access to money is very different. The police treated me and my family very different. The interference in your life is different. When I was young I went through juvenile court and it was so obvious that we were seen as scum, my parents, too. It was a kangaroo court. Later cops who busted my house, I was a piece of shit in their eyes. I mean really, who could I complain to if they treated me badly? I think they know this, too. Now it's different, but I never feel too safe. [Hope]

So right from the beginning ... I was found guilty of possession for the purpose [laughs] and so right from the beginning, the laws, I felt, were against me as a woman and as a poor woman and they were pro this guy who had the good lawyer and whose father had money. [Carol]

And I have grade school education. So, uhm ... I think that a lot of times, that people talk to me like I'm illiterate or something. Or couldn't make a conscious choice about anything, because I don't understand the issues involved. But I do understand my own life and my own needs very well. [Pat]

In contrast to women who are more visible and less protected in society

women who came from white, middle- and upper-class families were buf-
feted from many of the negative consequences of the law:

So, we got arrested together and because I come from a family where they're
white and I would say, middle class, with educational prestige, because it wasn't
that we had money but that there was the prestige of having a father who was
involved with the law and things like that ... that it was the first time I was aware of
the double standard, because the person I was with got sent to juvenile detention
and she wasn't even responsible. I mean, she wasn't even ... it was me that was
doing the whole trip ... So I was absolute, I was angry, I was dumbfounded. I
mean, certainly, part of me was relieved, 'cause I didn't have to go spend the
night in juvenile detention. But another part of me was just amazed, 'cause I had
never seen that distinction before. And to see how blatant it was, how incredibly
blatant the whole thing was. [Debbie]

Yeah, I was afraid I was going to go to jail with two little kids sitting outside, and if
my mother hadn't helped me with the money I would have gone to jail ... so I
mean, you're talking about women with money and women without money.
[Janet]

Out of maybe fifteen charges I spent three weeks in jail. I was lucky with my lawyers, because my family, when I was young, there was a lot of deaths in my family
with caretakers and stuff, because of that and because, I think partly because I
went to university. And I, it almost seemed like the lawyers would play, well the
last five or six years I had the same lawyer, sort of played with the mighty fallen
kind of thing. I got off easier, like I had struggled so hard and then fallen. When
actually, I don't know if I did struggle much. [Donna]

Because my husband kept me away from a lot of it. I would have either got into a
lot more trouble or I would have quit using if I hadn't been with him. But, I was
arrested for heroin, morphine a few times, and I didn't go to jail. I think that I
didn't go to jail because ... well, I was working and I was able to get recommendations and support. And because I knew how to present myself. So, I think absolutely that ... [class] makes a difference. [Diane]

Presenting oneself as a member of conventional society is paramount
when interacting with the criminal justice system. If the women could por-
tray themselves as middle-class, or upper-class, with social and financial
support, they discovered that the police used discretion, and the judges
were often sympathetic. Furthermore, past loss of child custody, single-

parent status, welfare-recipient status, and lengthy criminal records often were perceived by the criminal justice system as signs of deviance. The women, and especially women of colour, were punished. Poor women of European heritage were punished as well, and some of these women spoke about their belief that their sentencing was harsh because the judge wanted to make an example of them for transgressing into criminal behaviour. This was evident upon sentencing and parole hearings:

The parole board itself decided not to let me go, and they said the reason was my age, because I was thirty-two when it happened ... because ... I was white and I had more opportunities because I came from C. 'Cause I had every opportunity not to do it. And on the map C. is a rich area. It's a ridiculous system. It's very corrupt. And these few people look at your files and say who goes and who stays ... But they just said, 'We're giving you an eleven-month hit.' [Morgan]

White women do suffer persecution as illicit drug users, and it is safe to say that *all criminalized women* receive harsh treatment within the criminal justice system, especially women who are perceived as 'undeserving' (Edwards, 1987; Radford, 1987) But the institutionalization of racism has far-reaching effects for women of colour, and all of the other women interviewed claimed that women of colour had a more difficult time than they did in relation to police harassment, arrest, and sentencing.

Re-entry

The parole board plays a significant role in the release of women who are incarcerated. It is well documented that the National Parole Board has not been consistent in 'establishing clear and consistent criteria for release decisions' (Griffiths & Verdun-Jones, 1989, p. 452). The discretionary power of the National Parole Board has been problematic for many women hoping for release, including some of those interviewed for this study. One professional woman from working-class background noted:

I had no trouble with the law at all until ... ten years later, when I was a very casual user of hard drugs. I would say if I used once a month I would be ... I would worry that was too much [at the time of her arrest]. And ... so I just assumed I was going to get my parole and they turned me down. That was devastating to me. And I thought ... as a mother ... It had absolutely no meaning that I was a mother who had a relationship with this child and who ... had a really good plan on release. I think one of the reasons I never got it is that C. and I were still together. And because he was an addict, they looked at him and what he was doing, instead of looking at me and what I was doing. [Carol]

Another woman from a working-class background stated:

Oh, yeah, the other thing about the parole board, is when you go up before them ... they decide right then and there ... sometimes they decide before. But ... I heard this from the other inmates there, ... I don't know if this is true, if they think you are probably not going to commit another crime, if it's mostly then a one [time] thing, then they might keep you longer. Because I knew so many people who were in, you know, the revolving door, or recidivism. Where they are in and out, and in and out. In some instances they let them go because they know they are coming back. So they don't worry so much about it. Like, that's from an inmate point of view. And that's what they told. But I listened to the inmates because they know a lot, they really know about the system really well, plus it's the inmate point of view.

And so I thought about that and I thought that might be true because I knew, I knew I wasn't going to risk, I felt what happened to me ... You know, I didn't have a record, for one thing. I didn't have any record for ten years. Like I did stuff when I was younger and then I went through a long period of time when I didn't get in trouble ... and then they brought it up in court, the stuff that happened when I was a kid ... But they just said, We are giving you an eleven-month hit,' which meant I was doing eleven more months conditional time. Which was a big disappointment to me, and considering I had a child, and I tried to tell them, you know I had a child, a little four-year-old son.

... it's almost like you go into a dream because you know you have a chance to get out and you've done the best you can while you're in there, there's nothing more you can do ... what I did was a series of banks so they looked at every individual bank as a separate crime. So they said because there were so many ... [Morgan]

The women had hoped that their good behaviour and their status as mothers would be acknowledged by the parole board. But in fact their status as mothers, rather than compelling leniency, appeared to compel punitive decisions from the parole board. Similar to other research (see Carlen, 1983; Daly, 1989; Eaton, 1986; Masson, 1992), the women in this study believed they received more severe sentencing for failing to assume the proper gender role of the 'good mother.' The master status of 'criminal' overrides their status as 'mother' as women enter the criminal justice system (Faith, 1993).

For women whose partners were incarcerated, parole board decisions were also significant. One woman discussed her husband's difficulty in receiving parole:

But he's really quiet ... so ... one time he didn't get a parole ... And I see people out there also who, some of them ... they can't write ... and it's really hard. It's hard enough in society in general. Then you get a person who's coming up against the system, and it's really hard, you know. [Linda]

The parole board and the criminal justice system as a whole can be problematic for individuals who are not articulate or who cannot write well. This often has little to do with a lack of understanding on the part of the criminalized women; rather, the professionals they encounter treat them as inferior and incapable of making decisions pertaining to their sentencing and release. One woman on social assistance noted:

All through arrest, or court, or social workers ... All that stuff, they all go ahead and make all kinds of decisions without even consulting you or even letting you know that anything is in the process of being done. It just makes you feel like a rag doll ... It is so combative every time you try to open your mouth that after a while, you just say, 'Fuck, what is the point? Let these people do what they are going to do and I will just go on about my business and hope that they don't fuck with me too much.' [Pat]

Although drug treatment was not available to the women interviewed during their time in prison, some of them noted that it was difficult for drug users to be honest with prison staff about their drug use, especially since this may affect their parole:

Say for instance in prison, where people will go in and the ones that can express themselves will go up to counsellors, tell the counsellors just what they want to hear ... so they're afraid to be truly ... honest ... being in jail and you're a drug addict, well, 'When you get out are you going to use drugs?' Well ... in fact Brannon Lake had a questionnaire like that. What were your feelings. And if you say yes, they're going to know ... or you're going to say, 'No, I'm never gonna use.'..Well, you can't, because if you say no, you're never going to use drugs, they know you're lying. If you say yes, you're not going to get a parole. [Linda]

Women who use illicit drugs are often in a double bind when answering questions related to their drug use. Although many of the women knew they would return to either legal drug use, such as a methadone maintenance program, prescription drug use, or illicit drug use, abstinence was the required behaviour for release. Furthermore, illicit drugs are available in prison (Barry, 1992). One woman of European heritage noted that, while she was in jail, she was committed to abstinence due to the penalties for being caught:

I was institutionalized for so long, and I was basically away from drugs, although there was drugs in jail too. [Morgan]

Briton's (1995) study within the United Kingdom demonstrated that offenders are unwilling to share tales of drug misuse with probation officers due to their fear that they will lose more than they gain. 'At risk is their liberty, their sources of drugs, their relationships with parents and school, their children, their partners, and their jobs or welfare benefits' (Briton, 1995, p. 16). Canadian women are also reluctant to discuss their illicit drug use with criminal justice officials. One professional woman described her attempts to conceal her lifestyle from criminal justice officials when she was poor and on probation:

When I was on probation I never responded to any of the personal questions asked by the probation officer. I knew my private life would be seen as further evidence of my incorrigibility. And I was having a hell of a time just maintaining an acceptable social front at that time. [Hope]

The transition out of prison could be fraught with problems. Reunions with partners and children were sometimes happy moments. However, the long separation often traumatizes children, and mothers have to work on both their children's problems and their own upon release. Most of the women had not been offered counselling or drug treatment during their incarceration. Upon release they found many issues pertaining to their drug use and their status as criminalized women unresolved:

The jail wasn't set up at all to accommodate anybody that was doing any kind of long term, and there was no rehabilitation of any kind. They didn't have any counsellors that knew how to do any kind of therapy, that were, where I could gain any insight about myself. It was all just work on yourself. You know that isn't always successful. [Carol]

I spent time in jail for drug-related crimes ... A lot of problems just being in jail and then having to come back out. And that's going to be a lifelong thing for me because I still have a record. [Morgan]

Many of the women had taken initial steps to receive a pardon if they had only one or two criminal offences related to illicit drugs. One middle-class woman who had been convicted of a narcotic offence described the difficulty of obtaining a pardon:

No, I sent away for all the stuff for a pardon. I got the stuff back and ... I never took it past that point. I haven't got the pardon yet. You have to put down the names of two or three people that they can interview about you. Who can I ask? You would also have to know someone that you didn't mind knowing about your charges. Mind you, it was just marijuana, but even so. But that doesn't matter, it was a tiny little bit, it shows up as possession of narcotics. I could have just had a ton of cocaine or something like that. And now, I should really get that pardon, honestly. I started about two years ago and there my fingerprints sit ... So now I have to go through the whole ordeal again. And what ... was really frustrating was when I got my record back it showed that I had got a conditional discharge with probation, because it was a gram and a half of marijuana. But it didn't say that. It just said possession of narcotics. And when you get eighteen months suspended, I mean probation, you might think, God, this was really bad. But it wasn't, it was marijuana. On top of that ... when I got busted for shoplifting one time and I beat it. That was also down there. [Gloria]

The stigma attached to illicit drug use hinders women trying to re-enter conventional society. Many of the women interviewed had few friends or family members who would be eligible to be interviewed for the pardon. Often the people available had criminal records themselves, or lacked professional status. Looking outside their own circle of friends and family meant having to reveal their past, something that many of them were reluctant to do.

For women re-entering conventional society after release from prison, race and class were of primary importance. Poor women had little economic support. Women of colour had to face the same institutional and personal racism that accompanied them to prison. Having a criminal record made re-entry more difficult. One low-income woman spoke about the difficulty she had in finding employment. She noted that her visible prison tattoos on her hands, and her visibility as a women of Native Indian heritage, contributed to this difficulty:

I wanted to work with children ... So I went out ... I was so stupid, I went out to West Vancouver and I was going out to these rich people's places. Going for interviews. I sounded really nice on the phone and everything, but when I went there, you know, people saw that I was Native and got turned off. [Sue]

Women who were able to maintain a semblance of middle-class status were often able to hide their identity as criminalized women and drug users. Participation in a methadone program enabled one middle-class woman of European heritage to enrol in a graduate program and to re-enter society more easily than other women who had no access to education and social and economic supports:

I am sure that after university or anywhere I go, I am sure that nobody would be able to guess in a million years that I was on methadone. [Diane]

A successful re-entry into conventional society is obviously relevant to recidivism and stabilization. The availability of non-judgmental economic and social support is paramount.

The criminalization of specific drugs has made it difficult for women to re-enter mainstream society, for the social stigma continues long after one ceases illicit drug use and criminal activity. Criminal charges, social service intervention, child apprehensions by the Ministry of Social Services, medical records, school records, and physical scars can all become evidence which permits discrimination.

Many of the women described their painful attempts to re-enter mainstream society:

Coming back into your life and trying to put it back in order. Within the system it is so difficult ... maybe some other societies it wouldn't be looked upon as so awful, people can bounce back. But in our society there's no bouncing back, you are out. And if they don't do it to you, you do it to yourself. This has been my worst problem ... Where I have literally oppressed my own self. And I put myself down and said, 'Oh, no, I could never do that. No, I couldn't do that. Because I'm not, you know, because I'm so awful.' ... And I'm just starting to think I'm not awful, I'm not awful. You know, even if I said to myself I wouldn't hurt anybody. It's like ... the system has made me afraid of myself. And distrustful of myself. But I see with my children how much I love them, and how much my children love me, and my boyfriend and my family. And if my family loves me and my children love me I'm not so bad. I mean, who is the system talking to, who are they talking to, and where do they get their information from, and how do they impose their moral judgments upon others? [Morgan]

But, unfortunately, when you are trying to live within a system, and now ... I have made a decision that I am going to be part of that system, as far on the edge as I am. I think that it is a healthy fear, to be afraid of those things. To say who I really am. It is an ongoing struggle for me, though, for sure. [Carol]

I kicked that habit and I went on to get straight and ... and live normal or whatever that was. I got a job. I had my first kid, you know, a couple of years later ... But I felt ... it was really weird having to invent a past. I was pretty young still then in my twenties. And I had never been to high school. I had never been on a date. Had never done anything that most people that I was talking to were still talking about. And so I had to invent this past, which was really, really weird. [Pat]

For women who wish to be honest about their past and regain a sense of their own integrity, the stigma and legal sanctions surrounding illicit drug use make re-entry problematic. These women spoke about the oppression they experienced as women who have children:

As a matter of fact, even now I think that if I were a man, I would be a lot more comfortable to share my background and be accepted, but because I am a woman, I feel more pressure to hide that because it goes so against society's view of what a woman is supposed to do and who she is supposed to be in terms of nurturing and children and ... being the one that always is ... doing what she is supposed to do. I mean, I reject all of that. I think that it is a bunch of poop! But, unfortunately, when you are trying to live within a system ... [Carol]

Well, being a woman in itself, there's a lot of oppression in that sphere. We may not all see it, we may not be all willing to admit it, but I felt there's a lot of oppression in just being a woman. Especially being a woman with a low income. And then, you know, [oppression] by males, and if your self-esteem is low, the person you envision yourself with, once your self-esteem is at that low point, you don't, you just don't envision yourself with a college professor or a lawyer. You see yourself with, you know, someone who may be abusive to you and may be oppressive to you. So, it's just layers of oppression and repression. It happens to us, other people expect us to be this, and we become this, and we expect a little bit from ourselves. [Morgan]

Many of the women noted that their options were limited as women and as mothers. Their past was reflected in their present and future, and options were limited in their private and public lives. In addition, many of the women carry physical scars related to their past drug use. Abscesses, needle marks, and so on, are often difficult to hide:

This is a miss, on my arm, and on my hand the doctor had to cut that one, and this one is a miss too. This vein the centre vein, is all broken, there's no main vein here at all, this one is too calloused. [Jill]

There are some things about people that, sometimes, I can pick out the ex-users. There are certain body scars that just don't, will always ... [Pat]

Straight women like men who live a little dangerously, who have a past. You know, a tattoo looks okay on a guy, or a wild past. But for women who are trying to find a straighter life, their past is not looked on the same way. If a women has lost her kids, that's seen as horrible. If she has track marks, tattoos, this is not so attractive to straight people. [Morgan]

For women who have a past, especially a criminal past, body scars can signify criminal status (Faith, 1993) and complicate reintegration. Rosenbaum notes that women who have a history of illicit drug use are viewed as 'damaged goods' by society (1981, p. 132). Social attitudes dictate that a certain degree of deviant behaviour is tolerable in men, but women are punished for past transgressions:

We really judge women who use way more critically. But especially mothers, she is despised because drug use means you are a bad mother. But my feelings for my kids is the same as it was when I used. It hasn't changed. It angers me that women carry the brunt of these things. Men take such little responsibility for anything in our society. And raising kids on your own is difficult and the price of using drugs is so much higher for mothers. [Hope]

A woman's illicit drug use, and especially that of mothers, is regarded differently from male illicit drug use. Return to society is often perceived as conditional. One mother of two children who is working towards her university degree stated:

I feel like I just have something inside of me, and I've been allowed to bounce back. I've been allowed to. I am fighting back, but I've also been allowed to do that. Because they could have put me in jail forever, or I could have been refused welfare, or might not have been able to get my grants for school. [Morgan]

For many women, their criminalized status continues to affect their lives even after they stabilize and discontinue illicit drug use.

Criminalization, Decriminalization, and Legalization

The persecution of illicit drug users has been accompanied by stereotypical depictions of drug users by the media. Drug laws and the media's depiction of the dangerousness of illicit drug use often shapes societies view of who illicit drug users are. Many of the women interviewed discussed the negative media attention illicit drug use is given, as well as the glamorization of drug use. Another concern was the more aggressive war on drugs in the United States, and how Canada may be affected by U.S. policy:

If the propaganda changed then people's ideas would start changing. You know, if they start seeing the reality of what they are doing, the whole subculture they are making ... this desperate subculture, it's just craziness. [Janet]

There used to be more money spent on educating people with ... you know, reefer kind of madness. Kind of misinformation, dis-information. [Diane]

These insane images the media and government has created of drug dealers is just like the images they create of enemies during wars. It's pure propaganda. And look how the U.S. is combining those images with Noriega, the drug dealer, the enemy, which gave the U.S. the impetus to invade Panama. It's quite frightening. It is obvious that prohibition does not work. We saw that during alcohol prohibition, the laws created more harm, violence, black markets, and actually more consumption of alcohol. That is what is happening with drugs too. But we don't want to face this. I don't know if it is our close proximity to the states, but I wish we would develop something different. I mean, look at it there. But it's terrible here too. [Hope]

Yeah, I do think they should legalize it. I really do. I mean, its not going away. They are talking about the army going down to Colombia. I mean, it is just stupid, you know, in the States, it really doesn't make sense. It's like an industry now, there's this big industry that sucks off of drugs being criminalized. And the criminal element gains from it. And the police agents and the weapons manufacturers and all that, they benefit from it being illegal. But I mean. Keeping it illegal doesn't really make much sense. [Gloria]

When I started using I think one of the reasons, and now it seems ridiculous when I look back ... but I think I used because it was illegal ... and I really believe that if they decriminalized it, it would deglamorize it. And I think ... well, it's just not glamorous, but the media tend, even the police are affected by it ... I really believe if it had been legal, for me ... I wouldn't have. It was sort of like a no-no, the ultimate no-no. [Linda]

Other women spoke about the long-term effects of the criminalization of certain drugs, as well as their sense that they were not protected by the law in general. The drug laws affected both drug use and choice of drug, as well as lifestyle. Some of the women expressed a general weariness with the lifestyle:

I am just tired of the game, you know. I am tired of quitting, starting up again, getting really involved. This is a big circle. If they had left it legal, I probably to this day would be a chippy user. You know, semi-wired. But, I mean, probably lifelong. You know, but it probably would have been a fairly even use of drugs. Like, you know, somebody going out for a beer, and in the evening having a pipe of opium or whatever. I would have been happy as hell. Why people have to get involved and tell you this is wrong and my morals are all screwed up. Their morals are all fucking screwed up, man. They just, they damned near destroyed this family twice. [Theresa]

But maybe if the taboos were not so restrictive and if the legal position was changed and things are loosened up a little bit. Maybe that wouldn't happen, maybe that wouldn't be the inevitability of it. Maybe a person could, you know, like maybe they actually could be, because, you know, I smoke pot in a perfectly acceptable way to me. I can not smoke pot for six months and it doesn't bother me at all. And then I'll have a couple of tokes and have a really good time. I love it and that's the end of it. But it doesn't. I don't care. Once in a while I think, 'Oh I'd like a toke,' but it's more like 'I'd like a jelly doughnut, you know.' I mean it's not a big deal. [Gloria]

But most of all it was the fear, the worry, that I could be busted. At certain times I didn't worry, like when I was a kid. But as I got older it did worry me and I didn't want to live with that constant fear or harassment. I didn't want to be treated so cruelly either, by cops. [Hope]

Yes. I mean, there the law and the system is screwed ... Yeah, I mean everything is screwed. You know, the whole law sucks. I have no respect for the law. Why should I? Nothing has helped me in the past, you know. [Liz]

Other women discussed the health and moral issues surrounding which drugs are currently legal and illegal in Canada:

You know, what drugs are, these drugs are okay but those drugs aren't okay. And it's a moral issue. And okay, what if they made alcohol illegal like they did, would the price tend to go up? What if they make cigarettes twenty bucks a cigarette, which could happen. [Morgan]

I don't think the law ... you know, you can't, you can't legislate morality. [Linda]

I mean, it is out to lunch. I mean, this war on drugs ... they are letting out child abusers so that they can make room for all these addicts. The costs, I mean, it is just wild. If there are aliens out there, they must just think ... bizarre. [Diane]

Several of the women expressed their concern that the way professionals and society in general treated them influenced their options and responses. It is interesting to note that the majority of the women viewed their drug use as their own responsibility. Very few described their drug use in terms of the disease model. Drugs, both licit and illicit, could be used responsibly:

I'm not justified in doing that either [forgery], but the drugs didn't make me do it. I actually did that. But I, I don't, I just think I had a lot of anger. I had a lot of anger. [Morgan]

But, I mean ... like alcohol ... You have got to be responsible that you don't drink and drive and you have got be responsible how you take your alcohol. I think that would be the same thing for any drug. I mean, anybody can do drugs, responsibly or irresponsibly. Anybody can do it from a doctor today. You know, they can get their pills and their, you know, as prescribed or not. [Evelyn]

The majority of the women interviewed felt that drugs must be decriminalized in Canada:

I want all drugs legal. I am a total anti-prohibition ... You know ... laws against personal freedoms never worked. It is as simple as that. [Theresa]

I don't think any person should be penalized for drug use itself. That is not a crime, nor is buying it or selling it. We need to decriminalize drugs, to offer more organic drugs, opium, liquid cocaine, try to move away from the more potent pharmaceuticals. Try to re-establish drugs back into our society the way they were before these laws. Just a fact of life. [Hope]

Well, I think ... it should not be illegal. Addictions should not be illegal. It should not be illegal. I think it should be provided for us, whether we have to buy it through prescriptions or whatever. I think it should be decriminalized. [Diane]

I think the law is ... I think they've got to get it decriminalized. They certainly have to decriminalize marijuana and hashish and they have to decriminalize narcotics ... [Janet]

I think they have to legalize drugs ... I mean, I just think it is the sensible thing to do. [Gloria]

Many of the women recognized the need for dialogue about decriminalization; however, they did not want to reveal their own drug use for fear of arrest, loss of employment, and social alienation. One woman summed up a lot of the concerns surrounding illicit drug use – the stigmatization of use, the cost, the fear, and the need for open dialogue:

Because of the ways that the laws have gone, we see those people as bad ... we tend to ... like, as a society to blame them for the ills of society instead of understanding that ... if we considered decriminalizing everything, I mean ... to me, we would be much further ahead. I mean the government is spending millions and billions of dollars in North America on fighting a war, quote, that they all know that they're losing ... but, you see, it is not for even myself to speak out against ... to speak out against making more laws and making them stricter. It is ... you know, it is often hard to do that. I live in a really conservative province. And as a social worker, I want to be able to say those things, but I also worry that there will be ramifications if I do. So, I am very hesitant and I really feel out ... the group of people I am in, before I say what I really feel. But, I think that if everybody that felt, that was comfortable to start talking about it, that it might create a dialogue. I think that is what we need, Is to begin a dialogue. Because if people don't talk about it and talk about how they really feel, it will never change. [Carol]

Conclusion

Women who use illicit drugs are stigmatized and criminalized. Women of colour, poor women, and more visible users are the most vulnerable to arrest and police harassment. But few of the women interviewed, whether poor or middle-class, were able to escape acquiring a criminal record for drug and drug-related offences. With few economic options, women drift into drug dealing, prostitution, and other non-violent crimes to support their families and their illicit drug use. However, in contrast to media images of illicit drug users engaging in predatory illegal activity to support their drug use, the women interviewed also participated in legitimate part- and full-time employment and maintained ties to conventional society.

When women are released from prison, even if they have ceased their illicit drug use, re-entry into conventional society is often difficult. Stigma, criminal records, and temporary and permanent loss of children have far-reaching effects in terms of employment, future relationships, continued police surveillance and harassment, and subsequent problems associated with the loss of children. The women interviewed viewed mothering and family caretaking as their primary responsibilities, although their status as criminals overshadowed their status as mothers in the criminal justice system.

The criminalized status attached to women who use illicit drugs contributes to their lack of legitimacy and voice in Canadian society. The Controlled Drugs and Substances Act (previously the Narcotic Control Act) legitimizes punitive government and police activity that erodes civil liberties, and women (and men) are persecuted. The contradictions inherent in the Controlled Drugs and Substances Act are evident when the dangerousness of legal drugs such as alcohol and tobacco is examined. Tobacco and alcohol are our most dangerous drugs, but the Controlled Drugs and Substances Act maintains a social fiction relating to the 'dangerousness' of specific drugs. Although it is socially unacceptable for women to drink heavily and smoke tobacco during pregnancy in North America, the criminalization of women who use illicit drugs involves much heavier penalties.

Rather than the criminalization of drugs, what is needed, as one women stated, is 'dialogue.' This dialogue ought to focus the state's interest in prohibiting altered states of consciousness through drug legislation, and in the state's interest in blaming illicit drug use for society's social and economic problems. The continued criminalization of illicit drugs disregards the class, race, and gender issues underlying the enactment and enforcement of the Controlled Drugs and Substances Act. One woman warned:

And that as a society ... we should be frightened by it. By what we are doing with so many people. You know, it reminds me of the conservative time in history and how we have ... tended to isolate all those that don't fit in. [Carol]

Persecuting women (and men) who wish to alter their consciousness is cruel and counter-productive. Canada must search for more complex answers to its social and economic ills than the criminalization of narcotics and the race, class, and gender biases that underlie this criminalization.

7

Implications for Policy Makers

Our society suffers from a lack of information about women who use illicit drugs and the institutions that often define and shape their lives. The study discussed in this book derived from open-ended interviews with twenty-eight mothers in Western Canada in 1993–4 facilitated the airing of opinions on this important topic. It shows how the behaviour of mothers who use illicit drugs is regulated through formal and informal social controls and the impact of ideologies. The legal, medical, and social service professions in Canada control and punish these mothers. Current drug legislation and policy regarding illicit drug, especially by mothers, are based on ideologies concerning 'good and bad' drugs, familial ideology, and gender-specific roles for mothers,.

Policy Directions

Currently, women who use illicit drugs are perceived to be unfit mothers, and their children are judged by social workers to be at risk. Social workers often have little education about cultural differences, drug use, and alternative family formations. The Chief Coroner of B.C. (Cain, 1994) recently presented the concerns of provincial social workers in relation to working with women who use illicit drugs. Although this was not Cain's intention, the social workers' comments reveal their ignorance concerning drug use and mothering, as well as the lack of available services for women that are not threatening and judgmental. The social workers' underlying message was that all drug use is 'a child protection concern' and that, although numerous services are available to women who use illicit drugs, they refuse them (Cain, 1994, p. 39).

In the province of British Columbia, social workers and family court

judges were informed by Sunny Hill Hospital for Children about the supposed short- and long-term problems associated with neonatal abstinence
syndrome (NAS). Medical testimony from Sunny Hill has been utilized in
determining the outcomes of custody cases involving infants labelled with
NAS. The NAS program at Sunny Hill was the only one of its kind in the
province of British Columbia, and an opposing opinion was lacking; consequently, medical criteria developed by Sunny Hill were given more
weight than other information about the short- and long-term effects of
NAS.

There is no specific social service legislation in Canada that specifically
equates maternal drug use with neglect or child abuse. Nevertheless, as
demonstrated by the data presented in this study, children have been
apprehended by the Ministry of Social Services due to their mothers' illicit
drug use or past history of illicit drug use, and as the result of being
labelled with NAS. B.C.'s first Minister for Children and Families, Penny
Priddy, announced that the ministry has a new protocol (Protocol For
Cooperation between Staff of Ministry for Children and Families and Physicians) with the College of Physician and Surgeons outlining how information about mothers who are identified as illicit drug users will be shared
(McInnes, 1997). Although this new protocol only reinforces existing
policy, it may severely limit patient/doctor confidentiality (see Ministry for
Children and Families, 1997). The creation of the new ministry has already
been criticized, as it moves all alcohol and drug counsellors from the
Ministry of Health to the Ministry for Children and Families. Under the
new system, information about people going into drug treatment will be
shared with social services. This may prevent many mothers from obtaining help since social workers may perceive their illicit drug use as a child
protection concern (Ouston, 1997). Ouston (1997) states that this move
may have been a response to a few highly publicized cases in which it
appeared that parents who used illicit drugs harmed their children. But
more specifically, it is a response to a case in which a young First Nations
woman overdosed on heroin and her twenty-two-month-old son was left
alone with her body for several days. This case, coupled with the 1995 Gove
Report, which advocates child apprehension rather than the old social welfare policy of family reunification, has contributed to a climate of suspicion
and to the increasing regulation of mothers who use illicit drugs in B.C.

First Nations and poor women are overrepresented in terms of child
apprehension and the labelling of their children as having NAS. These
mothers' drug use is perceived as incompatible with good mothering,
and their children are judged to be at risk. The interests of child and

mother are portrayed as separate from each other. And the presumed interests of the child remain primary to social workers and family court judges, who have little direct experience with cultures of poverty. This has negative consequences for many women who come into contact with them. The identification of NAS as a 'high risk' medical problem has led to further intervention by these professionals, with little support for either mothers or children.

Illicit drug use does not equal poor parenting any more than does licit drug use. Whether they use illicit drugs or not, women are not traditionally offered extra services until family break-up occurs. When extra services or support are available, they are often delivered in a judgmental fashion and accompanied by thinly veiled surveillance. Furthermore, social workers often fail to recognize cultural differences and therefore strive to have women reject 'the day-to-day support network of friends and replace it with anonymous and distant, paid helpers' (Cain, 1994, p. 39).

The current surveillance of and intervention into the lives of poor women and women of colour is unwarranted. As long as social workers and social policy identify illicit drug use and other behaviour that fails to conform to traditional female gender roles as deviant, women and children will suffer. What is needed is non-judgmental social and economic support (similar to what foster parents receive), not surveillance and punishment.

The infants of women who use illicit drugs during pregnancy are defined as a challenge to the medical and social service professions. The medical community claims legitimacy and expertise in treating neonatal abstinence syndrome and looking after maternal health. In response to maternal illicit drug use, the medical community has created regimens of care that focus on managing individual women and their infants.

Illicit drug use is only one of many factors influencing maternal outcomes. Legal drugs – alcohol and tobacco – are more widely used and appear to be more dangerous to infants than illegal drugs. Yet researchers and maternal and infant programs continue to focus on the use of illicit drugs. Like the consequences of illicit drug use for mothers, the labelling of infants as having NAS is mediated by the mothers' race and class. To date, outside of infant withdrawal, all short- and long-term NAS symptoms are unsubstantiated. Infant withdrawal from prenatal exposure to opiate derivatives ranges from mild to severe, and is unpredictable and transitory.

Women who use illicit drugs are held personally responsible for the outcomes of their pregnancies, regardless of social environments that may negatively affect pregnancy outcomes and mothering in general.

The medical community in North America views the ideal pregnancy as drug free, unless the drugs are clinically prescribed. The social stigma surrounding maternal drug use takes a personal toll on women. Women drug users, and especially mothers who use drugs, are viewed as more deviant than their male counterparts, and this stereotype contributes to their silencing and lack of legitimacy. In contrast to the Sunny Hill experiment, programs in England and Scotland strongly suggest that women's social and economic environment shapes maternal health. When women are offered non-judgmental midwifery services and social and economic support, maternal outcomes are similar to those seen in non-drug-using mothers.

The debates surrounding maternal drug use reveal the differences and assumptions underlying two models of health: the medical model and the social model. According to the medical model of health, pregnancy and birth are a medical problem requiring medical intervention in order to decrease risk (Wagner, 1994). The social model of health perceives birth as a biosocial process that is part of the fabric of daily life. It takes into consideration social factors that affect maternal outcomes, such as poverty, poor nutrition, and lack of support. Maternal services for women who use illicit drugs should strive to normalize pregnancy and birth and to provide services that meet the needs of the mothers.

Conclusion

Policy makers and medical, social service, and legal professionals need to be exposed to alternative views of illicit drug use and, in particular, maternal drug use. Women in general need to have access to information concerning maternal drug use that is factual rather than alarmist.

In North America the label NAS is a cultural construct that serves the medical, social service, and legal professions by facilitating increased social control of women. 'High risk' labels and legal, medical, and social service interventions serve to separate families and to stigmatize and punish both infant and mother. Social attitudes towards mothers who use illicit drugs have implications for all women, especially when maternal drug use is presented as so 'dangerous' that intervention by the state and medical agencies is considered worthy, even when such intervention undermines civil liberties in the most fundamental manner.

Current practices of social control of mothers who use illicit drugs – including coerced medical intervention, new and extended legal and civil liabilities, and child protection and welfare obligations – create categories of regulation that are gender-specific. These interventions have been recognized by the Royal Commission on New Reproductive Technologies (1993) as infringing on women's Charter rights. And recently the Supreme Court of Canada ruled that pregnant women cannot be detained and forced to undergo medical treatment against their will.

Nevertheless, liberal and conservative paradigms dominate the discussion of maternal drug use. Conservative researchers are quite biased and favour stringent legal sanctions, whereas liberal researchers offer logical arguments that appear to present both sides of the issue. Mothers are often absent from the discussion, which focuses on the foetus and on foetal harm. When mothers are included, their failure to mother is emphasized, and regulations and legal sanctions have been suggested to curb their behaviour. In addition, conservative fiscal policy and cutbacks in social and economic services have led politicians and professionals to look for simple answers to complex problems. Liberal and conservative paradigms limit the questions asked and the areas researched, ignoring and obscuring deeper issues of social control, gender, class, and race. One must question the medical, scientific, legal, and social service communities' interest in the developing foetus and in mothers who use illicit drugs. Their assumption that this interest benefits society is suspect.

Stanley Cohen states that 'every form of social control, actual or idealized, embodies a moral vision of what should be' (1985, p. 204). He concludes that we never fear too much control; rather, we fear too much chaos. However, control never works, for it leads to more control (Cohen, 1985, p. 235). The social control of mothers who use illicit drugs is driven by faulty ideologies that we embrace concerning illicit drugs, mothering, the family, and race, class, and gender. In our rush to blame and punish individual mothers who use illicit drugs, we fail to examine ideologies that are reflected in policy and law. Policy and emerging legislation constructed to regulate women who use illicit drugs contribute to and increase the social control and subordination of all women.

Policy and legislation concerning women and illicit drugs assume that there is only one family form – the nuclear family; that there is only one standard of mothering – white and middle class; that pregnancy and birth are medical rather than social events; that illicit drugs are more dangerous and compelling than licit drugs; that all women who use illicit drugs engage in other illegal acts and belong to marginal minority groups that are socially and economically deprived; that all women who use illicit drugs lie and manipulate; that the children of women who use illicit drugs are at risk due to maternal exposure to illicit drug use and parental abuse; and that women cannot regulate their illicit drug use. The study discussed in this book challenges these assumptions.

The marginalization of women who use illicit drugs, and of their children, reduces these women's ability to maintain a stake in conventional society. The increased number of women in prison for illicit drug charges in the United States, along with policies that encourage child apprehension in both the United States and Canada, can only lead to significant family disruption and the increased regulation of women. Illicit drug use, or drug use in itself, is a social problem that cannot be curtailed by harsh laws, incarceration, and mandatory drug treatment. Present and proposed methods of social control of mothers who use illicit drugs will only compound the problems that poor and minority women face today. Legalization of drugs would eliminate stigmatization, sentencing, and prison terms related to drug offences.

This study suggests that there is, in fact, a diverse group of women who use illicit drugs, in terms of age, race, and class. Aside from their shared status as mothers and their use of illicit drugs, the women interviewed were not a homogeneous group. The consequences of their illicit drug use were mediated by social status, race, class, gender, and social environment, as well as by the legal, social service, and medical communities. First Nations and poor women were overrepresented in terms of medical intervention, arrest, and child apprehension.

Women in Western society have witnessed social service, legal, and medical regulation during the last century. The punishment and regulation of pregnant women suspected of illicit drug use will not be restricted to only this small population; all women will be affected. Sheila Kitzinger notes that 'every society regulates the right to motherhood and "selects" those women who are allowed to be mothers' (1992, p. 17). In Canada, as elsewhere, women are often denied the chance to mother and raise their own children. The combination of our fear of illicit drugs, moralism, the regulation of reproduction, the suspected breakdown of the family and of traditional gender roles, racism, sexism, and classism has contributed to the social construction of mothers who use illicit drugs as scapegoats who embody all that is feared and considered evil in Western society. It would be to Canada's benefit to distance ourselves from policy which continues to extend the arm of the law to punish women who are suspected of illicit drug use. It is necessary to grant the illicit drug user adulthood, full rights, and some degree of expert status in relation to her own drug use. Only then will drug policy and drug treatment benefit the illicit drug user, her children, and society.

Interview Schedule

1. How did you get into using drugs (including alcohol)?
2. How has the criminalization of narcotics (the law) effected your life as a mother with children?
3. How did (or does) social services affect your life as a mother with children? ie. through intervention or apprehensions
4. Were any of your children labelled NAS or FAS?
   a. Did your child go to Sunny Hill?
   b. Or somewhere else?
   c. How were you and your infant treated?
5. If you had an audience of judges, social workers, police, what would you like to say to them about the law, social services, or just about your life as a mother who used drugs?
6. Do you think drug and alcohol treatment is effective? If so what kind do you think would work? If not, why?
7. Are you more worried about the narcotic laws or social services (apprehension)?
8. Has it been different for you being a mother who uses drugs than, say, a male drug user?
9. Have you been treated differently because of your class, race, or ethnicity by professionals in the criminal justice system (police, judges, probation officers, lawyers), social services, or the medical profession?
10. Has there been anything positive about your drug use?
11. What do you see in the future for yourself and your children?
12. Is there anything else that you would like to add?

Notes

Chapter 1: A Gender Analysis

1 The nuclear family is perceived as the basic family form in society. '"The family" is presented both in law and in popular culture as the basic unit in society, a sacred, timeless and so natural an institution that its definition is self-evident. Its privacy is sought to be protected and its sanctity proclaimed ... The ideal family, despite the gender-neutral references to "spouse" and "parent" in legislation, is still taken to mean a social relationship, sanctioned by law and preferably by religion, comprising a male adult, female adult, and their biological or adopted children' (Gavigan, 1988, p. 293).

2 The term 'ethnography' refers to the methodological approach developed by sociologists and anthropologists. Ethnographic sociological studies on illicit drug use seek to study the illicit drug user 'from within their culture rather than from outside it and to present their world as they see it' (Waldorf et al., 1991, p. 14). The concept of 'career' employed by ethnographic sociological studies 'makes it possible to look processually, sequentially, temporally, social psychologically, and (as much as possible), nonjudgmentally at the individual's experience with drugs (or any other type of career)' (Rosenbaum, 1981, p. 9). Traditionally, ethnographic sociological studies are based on participant observation and in-depth interviews.

3 'The meanings and practices of motherhood vary enormously through history, across cultures, and within the same culture – indicating that these "natural" realms of human experience are incessantly mediated by social praxis and design' (Petchesky, 1990, p. 9). By 'depicting motherhood as natural, a patriarchal ideology of mothering locks women into biological reproduction, and denies them identities and selfhood outside mothering' (Glenn, 1994, p. 9).

4 Familial ideology privileges the white, middle-class, nuclear family form in

both Canadian law and social policy within the 'private sphere' (Gavigan, 1988).

5 Canadian Charter of Rights and Freedoms, Part I of the Constitution Act, 1982.

6 Numerous ethnographic sociological studies of illicit drug use are available. See A. Lindesmith, 1947; H.S. Becker, 1953; and E. Preble and J.J. Casey, 1969. For more recent research see C. Faupel, 1991, and D. Waldorf, C. Reinarman, and S. Murphy, 1991. Other ethnographies of illicit drug use specific to women include M. Rosenbaum, 1981; A. Taylor, 1993; and L. Maher, 1995.

7 'Visible users' refers to those women whose illicit drug use was known to social service and legal professionals. 'Non-visible users' refers to women whose illicit drug use was not apparent to such professionals. Visibility does not remain static; many of the women were not visible users at the time of the interview but had been in the past, when they were on social assistance or in contact with the criminal justice system. However, not all of the women who had ceased to use illicit drugs were successful in becoming less 'visible.' Factors that determine visibility include successful re-entry into conventional society.

8 DAMS was a non-discriminatory group of women who met to offer support to each other. Their format was an alternative to NA and AA DAMS was dedicated to harm reduction, self-empowerment, and helping to meet the needs of women and their dependants. Women self-referred to DAMS, or were referred by other agencies. The majority of participants were from the Downtown Eastside of Vancouver, and most were mothers.

9 Alexander introduces the term 'continuum of involvement' to describe patterns of drug use. These include abstinence, experimental use, circumstantial use, casual use, regular recreational use, dependence, and addiction (1990, pp. 103, 104). Drug use is not static, and individuals can move within the continuum. Dependence refers to 'diminished flexibility' towards a specific drug. Overwhelming involvement distinguishes addictive use from dependent use. Alexander states that 'dependence may remain in the background of a person's life, but addiction is necessarily central and supplants other important activities' (1990, p. 105).

10 The quotations presented throughout this book have not been altered in terms of style of speech. Fictional names are used to preserve the anonymity of all the mothers interviewed.

Chapter 2: Drugs and Mothering

1 Throughout this book I refer to 'middle- and upper-class' users and 'poor' users. 'Poor users' refers to women who are visible illicit drug users on social

assistance. 'Middle- and upper-class users' refers to women who work or go to school.

Chapter 3: Neonatal Abstinence Syndrome (NAS): Sunny Hill Hospital for Children

1 See chapter 1 for a discussion on reproductive autonomy, and the medical model and social model of health.
2 Throughout this text the coding number [1] refers to the founding director of the Sunny Hill NAS program in Vancouver, British Columbia.

Chapter 5: Drug Treatment

1 Addiction: 'a behavioral pattern of drug use, characterized by overwhelming involvement with the use of a drug' (Jaffe, 1985, p. 533).

Chapter 6: The Effects of the Criminalization of 'Narcotics'

1 Canada's new drug law, the Controlled Drugs and Substance Act, prohibits the possession of cannabis products with a maximum penalty of five years less a day (Canada, 1996).

References

Acker, D., Sachs, B.P., & Tracey, K.J. (1983). Abruptio placenta associated with cocaine use. *American Journal of Gynaecology, 146*, 220–221.

Acker, J., Barry K., & Esseveld, J. (1991). Objectivity and truth. In M. Fonow & J. Cook (Eds.), *Beyond methodology* (pp. 133–153). Chicago: Aldine.

Addiction Research Foundation. (1994). *Gender issues in addictions research.* Toronto: Author.

Addiction Research Foundation. (1996). *The hidden majority.* Toronto: Author.

Addiction Research Foundation. (1997). Solvent's effect on fetus unproven. *The Journal, 26*(1), 2.

Adelberg, E., & Currie, C. (1993). Introduction. In E. Adelberg & C. Currie (Eds.), *In conflict with the law* (pp. 11–30). Vancouver: Press Gang.

Albersheim, S. (1994, June). Practical management of infants of substance-using mothers, and their long-term followup. In *Effects of alcohol and other drugs in pregnancy: Issues for families and communities,* Speaker Materials for a Conference to Address FAS and NAS, Vancouver, BC: Sunny Hill Health Centre for Children & Division of Continuing Education in the Health Sciences, The University of British Columbia (pp. 151–167).

Alexander, B. (1990). *Peaceful measures: Canada's way out of the 'War on Drugs.'* Toronto: University of Toronto Press.

Alexander, B., Beyerstein, B., & MacInnes, T. (1987). Methadone treatment in British Columbia: Bad medicine? *Canadian Medical Association Journal, 136*(1), 25–28.

Alexander, B., & Hadaway, P. (1981). Theories of opiate addiction: Time for pruning. *Journal of Drug Issues, 11*(1), 77–91.

Alexander, B., Hadaway, P., & Coambs, R. (1988). Rat Park chronicle. In J. Blackwell & P. Erickson (Eds.), *Illicit drugs in Canada* (pp. 63–68). Toronto: Methuen.

Almonte, B. (1994). Professionalization as culture change: Issues for infant/family community workers and their supervisors. *Zero to Three, 15*(2), 18–23.

Amir, D., & Biniamin, O. (1992). Abortion approval as a ritual of symbolic control. In C. Feinman (Ed.), *The criminalization of a woman's body* (pp. 5–25). New York: Harrington Park.

Arnup, K. (1994). *Education for motherhood: Advice for mothers in twentieth-century Canada.* Toronto: University of Toronto Press.

Ashbrook, D., & Solley, L. (1979). *Women and heroin abuse: A survey of sexism in drug abuse administration.* Palo Alto, CA: R & E. Research Associates.

Barry, E. (1992). Pregnant, addicted and sentenced: Debunking the myths of medical treatment in prison. *California Advocates for Pregnant Women, 19,* 1, 6, 7.

Becker, H.S. (1953). Becoming a marijuana user. *American Journal of Sociology, 59,* 235–242.

Becker, H.S. (1963). *Outsiders: Studies in the sociology of deviance,* Glencoe, IL: Free Press.

Bepko, C. (1991). *Feminism and addiction.* New York: Haworth.

Bernardi, E., Jones, M., & Tennant, C. (1989). Quality of parenting in alcoholics and narcotic addicts. *British Journal of Psychiatry, 154,* 677–682.

Beyerstein, B., & Hadaway, P. (1990). On avoiding folly. *Journal of Drug Issues, 20*(4), 689–700.

Biernacki, P. (1986). *Pathways from heroin addiction: Recovery without treatment.* Philadelphia: Temple University Press.

Binion, V. (1982). Sex differences in socialization and family dynamics of female and male heroin users. *Journal of Social Issues, 38*(2), 43–57.

Blackwell, J. (1983). Drifting, controlling and overcoming: Opiate users who avoid becoming chronically dependent. *Journal of Drug Issues, 13*(2), 219–235.

Bloom, B., Chesney-Lind, M., & Owen, B. (1994). Women in California prisons: Hidden victims of the war on drugs. In The Drug Policy Foundation (Ed.), *The crucial next stage: Health care & human rights* (Section G: 1–10). Washington, DC: Author.

Blume, S. (1992). Alcohol and other drug problems in women. In J. Lowinson, P. Ruiz, R. Millman, & J. Langrod (Eds.), *Alcohol and other drug problems in women* (pp. 794–807). Baltimore, MD: Williams & Wilkins.

Boer, K., & Kreyenbroek, M. (1989). Drug abuse in pregnancy. *International Planned Parenthood Federation Medical Bulletin, 23*(4), 1–3.

Bourne, R., & Newberger, E.H. (Eds.). (1979). *Critical perspectives on child abuse.* Lexington, MA: Lexington Books.

Boyd, N. (1983). The dilemma of Canadian narcotics legislation: The social control of altered states of consciousness. *Contemporary Crises, 7,* 257–269.

Boyd, N. (1984). The origins of Canadian narcotics legislation: The process of criminalization in historical context. *Dalhousie Law Journal, 8,* 102–136.

Boyd, N. (1990). *Criminological perspectives on social problems: Study guide.* Burnaby, BC: Centre for Distance Education, Simon Fraser University.

Boyd, N. (1991). *High society: Legal and illegal drugs in Canada.* Toronto: Key Porter.

Boyd, S.B. (1997). Challenging the public/private divide: An overview. In S.B. Boyd (Ed.), *Challenging the public/private divide: Feminism, law, and public policy* (pp. 3–33).

Brazelton, T., & Cramer, B. (1990). *The earliest relationship.* New York: Addison-Wesley.

Brecher, E., & The Editors of *Consumer Reports.* (1972). *Licit & illicit drugs.* Boston: Little, Brown.

Briton, C. (1995). Mind your own business. *Druglink, 10*(1), 16–17.

Brodie, H., & Thompson, J. (1981). The maximin strategy in modern obstetrics. *Journal of Family Practice, 12,* 977–986.

Brodie, J., Gavigan, S.A.M., & Jenson, J. (1992). *The politics of abortion.* Toronto: Oxford University Press.

Brooks v. Canada Safeway Ltd, (1989). S.C.R 1219, 59 D.L.R. (4th) 321.

Brown, E., & Zuckerman, B. (1991). The infant of the drug-abusing mother. *Pediatric Annals, 20*(10), 555–559, 581–583.

Burtch, B. (1994). *Trials of labour.* Montreal: McGill-Queen's University Press.

Cain, J. (1994). *Report on the Task Force into Illicit Narcotic Overdose Deaths in British Columbia.* Victoria, BC: Ministry of the Attorney General.

Callahan, J., & Knight, J. (1992). Prenatal harm as child abuse? In C. Feinman (Ed.), *The criminalization of a woman's body* (pp. 127–155). New York: Harrington Park.

Canada. 1995. Statutes of Canada. *Narcotic Control Act.* R.S., c. N-1, ss. 1, 4(3), 5(2), 8, 10, 16(2).

Canada. 1996. Statutes of Canada. *Controlled Drugs and Substance Act.* 45 Eliz., 2, c. 19.

Carlen, P. (1976). *Magistrates' justice.* London: Martin Robertson.

Carlen, P. (1983). *Women's imprisonment.* London: Routledge.

Centre for Reproductive Law & Policy (1996, February). Punishing women for their behavior during pregnancy. Fact sheet. New York: Author.

Chasnoff, I. (1988a). Drug use in pregnancy: Parameters of risk. *Pediatric Clinics of North America, 35*(6), 1403–1412.

Chasnoff, I. (1988b). Newborn infants with drug withdrawal symptoms. *Pediatrics in Review, 9*(9), 273–277.

Chasnoff, I. (1989). Cocaine, pregnancy, and the neonate. *Women & Health, 15*(3), 23–35.

Chasnoff, I., Burns, W., Schnoll, S., & Burns, K. (1985). Cocaine use in pregnancy. *New England Journal of Medicine, 313*(11), 664–669.

Chasnoff, I., Griffith, D., Freier, C., & Murray, J. (1992). Cocaine/polydrug use in pregnancy: Two-year follow-up. *Pediatrics, 89*(2), 337–339.

Chasnoff, I., Harvey, M., Landress, H., & Barrett, M. (1990). The prevalence of illicit-drug use or alcohol during pregnancy and discrepancies in mandatory reporting in Pinellas County, Florida. *New England Journal of Medicine, 322*(17), 1202–1206.

Chavkin, W. (1992). Women and fetus: The social construction of conflict. In C. Feinman (Ed.), *The criminalization of a woman's body* (pp. 193–202). New York: Harrington Park.

Chavkin, W., Allen, M., & Oberman, M. (1991). Drug abuse and pregnancy: Some questions on public policy, clinical management, and maternal and fetal rights. *Birth, 18*(2), 107–112.

Cheung, Y., Erickson, P., & Landau, T. (1991). Experience of crack use: Findings from a community-based sample in Toronto. *Journal of Drug Issues, 21*(1), 121–140.

Chunn, D. (1995). Feminism, law, and public policy: 'Politicizing the personal.' In N. Mandell & A. Duffy (Eds.), *Canadian families* (pp. 177–210). Toronto: Harcourt Brace.

Chunn, D., & Gavigan, S. (1991). Women and crime in Canada. In M. Jackson & C. Griffiths (Eds.), *Canadian criminology* (pp. 275–314). Toronto: Harcourt Brace Jovanovich.

Chunn, D., & Menzies, R. (1990). Gender, madness and crime: The reproduction of patriarchal and class relations in a psychiatric court clinic. *Journal of Human Justice, 1*(2), 33–54.

Clarke, J. (1996). The historical context of medicalization and gender: Its relationship to alcohol and other drug use in Canada. In M. Adrian, C. Lundy, & M. Eliany (Eds.), *Women's use of alcohol, tobacco and other drugs in Canada* (pp. 14–20). Toronto: Addiction Research Foundation.

Cohen, S. (1985). *Visions of social control.* Cambridge: Polity.

Collins, P. (1994). Shifting the center: Race, class, and feminist theorizing about mothering. In E. Glenn, G. Chang, & L. Forcey (Eds.), *Mothering: ideology, experience, and agency* (pp. 45–65). New York: Routledge.

Colten, M. (1980). A comparison of heroin-addicted and nonaddicted mothers: Their attitudes, beliefs, and parenting experiences. In *Heroin-addicted parents and their children: Two reports.* (National Institute on Drug Abuse Services Research Report, pp. 1–18). Washington, DC: U.S. Department of Health and Human Services; Public Health Service; Alcohol, Drug Abuse, and Mental Health Administration.

Colten, M. (1982). Attitudes, experiences, and self-perceptions of heroin-addicted mothers. *Journal of Social Issues, 38*(2), 77–92.

Cooperstock, R., & Hill, J. (1982). *The effects of tranquillization: Benzodiazepine use in Canada.* Ottawa: Health and Welfare Canada.

Cuskey, W.R. (1982). Female addiction: A review of the literature. *Journal of Addictions and Health, 72*, 1752–1769.

Daly, K. (1987). Structure and practice of familial-based justice in a criminal court. *Law & Society Review, 21*(2), 267–290.

Daly, K. (1989). Criminal justice ideologies and practices in different voices: Some feminist questions about justice. *International Journal of the Sociology of Law, 17*(1), 1–18.

Davin, A. (1978). Imperialism and motherhood. *History Workshop, 5*, 9–65.

Dembo, R., Williams, L., Wish, E., Berry, E., Getreu, A., Washburn, M., & Schmeidler, J. (1990). Examination of the relationships among drug use, emotional/psychological problems, and crime among youths entering a juvenile detention center. *International Journal of the Addictions, 25*(11), 1301–1340.

Densen-Gerber, J., & Rohrs, C. (1973). Drug-addicted parents and child abuse. *Contemporary Drug Problems, 2*(4), 683–695.

Dole, V. (1987). Methadone treatment in British Columbia: Bad medicine? *Canadian Medical Association Journal, 136*(8), 798.

Dole, V., & Nyswander, M. (1965). A medical treatment for diacetylmorphine (heroin) addiction: A clinical trial with methadone hydrochloride, *Journal of the American Medical Association, 193*, 646–650).

Dreher, M., Nugent, J., & Hudgins, R. (1994). Prenatal marijuana exposure and neonatal outcomes in Jamaica: An ethnographic study. *Pediatrics, 93*(2), 254–260.

Dunlap, E., & Johnson, B. (1996). Family and human resources in the development of a female crack-seller career: Case study of a hidden population. *Journal of Drug Issues, 26*(1), 175–198.

Dunlap, E., Johnson, B., & Maher, L. (1997). Female crack sellers in New York City: Who they are and what they do. *Women & Criminal Justice, 8*(4), 25–55.

Eaton, M. (1983). Mitigating circumstances: Familiar rhetoric. *International Journal of the Sociology of Law, 11*, 385–400.

Eaton, M. (1985). Documenting the defendant: Placing women in social inquiry reports. In J. Brophy & C. Smart (Eds.), *Women-in-law* (pp. 117–139). London: Routledge & Kegan Paul.

Eaton, M. (1986). *Justice for women? Family, court and social control.* Milton Keynes: Open University Press.

Edwards, A. (1987). Male violence in feminist theory: An analysis of the changing conceptions of sex/gender violence and male dominance. In J. Hanmer & M. Maynard (Eds.), *Women, violence and social control* (pp. 13–29). London: Macmillan.

Edwards, A. (1988). *Regulation and repression.* Sydney, Australia: Allen & Unwin.

Edwards, S. (1981). *Female sexuality and the law.* Oxford: Martin Robertson.

Ehrenreich, B., & English, D. (1973). *Witches, midwives, and nurses.* Feminist Press.

Erickson, P., Adlaf, E., Murray, G., & Smart, R. (1987). *The steel drug: Cocaine in perspective.* Toronto: Lexington Books.

Erickson, P., Riley, D., Cheung, Y., & O'Hare, P. (1997). *Harm reduction: A new direction for drug policies and programs.* Toronto: University of Toronto Press.

Erickson, P., & Watson, V. (1990). Women, illicit drugs, and crime. In L. Kozlowski, H. Annis, H. Cappell, F. Glaser, M. Goodstadt, Y. Israel, H. Kalant, E. Sellers, & E. Vingilis (Eds.), *Research advances in alcohol and drug problems* (Vol. 10, pp. 251–272). New York: Wiley.

Ettorre, E. (1992). *Women and substance use.* New Brunswick, N.J.: Rutgers University Press.

Faith, K. (1993). *Unruly women: The politics of confinement and resistance.* Vancouver: Press Gang.

Faupel, C. (1991). *Shooting dope: Career patterns of hard-core heroin users.* Gainesville: University of Florida Press.

Fields, A., & Walters, J. (1985). Hustling: Supporting a heroin habit. In B. Hanson et al. (Eds.), *Life with heroin: Voices from the inner city* (pp. 49–73). Toronto: Lexington Books.

Fingarette, H. (1994). We should reject the disease model. In B. Slife (Ed.), *Taking sides: Clashing views on controversial psychological issues* (8th ed. pp. 206–210). Guilford, CT: Dushkin Publishing Group.

Finnegan, L. (1979). *Drug dependence in pregnancy: Clinical management of mother and child.* (USDHEW publication N. ADM 79-678). Rockville, MD: U.S. Dept. of Health Education and Welfare, National Institute on Drug Abuse.

Fitzgerald, R. (1993). *Constructing 'fetal personhood' in the press: A study of the* Vancouver Sun*'s coverage of reproduction from 1969–1989.* Unpublished master's thesis, Simon Fraser University, Burnaby, BC.

Flagler, E., Baylis, F., & Rodgers, S. (1997). Bioethics for clinicians: 12. Ethical dilemmas that arise in the care of pregnant women: Rethinking 'maternal-fetal conflicts.' *Canadian Medical Association Journal, 156*(12), 1729–1732.

Frank, D., & Zuckerman, B. (1993). Children exposed to cocaine prenatally: Pieces of the puzzle. *Neurotoxicology and Teratology, 15,* 298–300.

Fricker, H., & Segal, S. (1978). Narcotic addiction, pregnancy, and the newborn. *American Journal of Diseases in Children, 132*(4), 360–366.

Fulroth, R., Phillips, B., & Durand, D. (1989). Perinatal outcome of infants exposed to cocaine and/or heroin in utero. *American Journal of Diseases in Children, 143,* 905–910.

Gallagher, J. (1987). Eggs, embryos and foetuses: Anxiety and the law. In M. Stanworth (Ed.), *Reproductive technologies* (pp. 139–150). London: Polity.

Gallagher, J. (1989). Fetus as patient. In S. Cohen & N. Taub (Eds.), *Reproductive laws for the 1990s* (pp. 185–235). Clifton, NJ: Humana.

Gavigan, S. (1988). Law, gender and ideology. In A. Bayefshy (Ed.), *Legal theory meets legal practice* (pp. 283–295). Edmonton: Academic Printing and Publishing.

Gavigan, S. (1992). *Paradise lost, paradox revisited: The implications of familial ideology for feminist, lesbian and gay engagement to law.* Unpublished manuscript, Osgoode Hall Law School, York University, North York, ON.

Gavigan, S. (1993). Women's crime: New perspectives and old theories. In E. Adelberg & C. Currie (Eds.), *In conflict with the law* (pp. 215–234). Vancouver: Press Gang.

Gieringer, D. (1990). How many crack babies? *The Drug Policy Letter, 11*(2), 4–5.

Glaser, B., & Strauss, A. (1967). *The discovery of grounded theory: Strategies for qualitative research.* Chicago: Aldine.

Glenn, E. (1994). Social constructions of mothering: A thematic overview. In E. Glenn, G. Chang, & L. Forcey (Eds.), *Mothering: Ideology, experience, and agency* (pp. 1–29). New York: Routledge.

Goldstein, P. (1979). *Prostitution and drugs.* Toronto: Lexington Books.

Gómez, L. (1994). *Processing and managing social problems: The institutionalization of pregnant women's drug use in the California legislature and criminal justice system.* Unpublished doctoral dissertation, Stanford University, Stanford, CA.

Goode, S. (1994). Heroin use and pregnancy. *Druglink, 9*(4), 13.

Gordon, L. (1990). Family violence, feminism, and social control. In L. Gordon (Ed.), *Women, the state, and welfare* (pp. 178–198). Madison: University of Wisconsin Press.

Gorlick, C. (1995). Divorce: Options available, constraints forced, pathways taken. In N. Mandell & A. Duffy (Eds.), *Canadian families* (pp. 211–234). Toronto: Harcourt Brace.

Graham, K., & Koren, G. (1991). Characteristics of pregnant women exposed to cocaine in Toronto between 1985 and 1990. *Canadian Medical Association Journal, 144*(5), 563–568.

Granfield, R., & Cloud, W. (1996). The elephant that no one sees: Natural recovery among middle-class addicts. *Journal of Drug Issues, 26*(1), 45–61.

Green, M. (1986). A history of Canadian narcotics control: The formative years. In N. Boyd (Ed.), *The social dimensions of law* (pp. 24–40). Scarborough, ON: Prentice-Hall.

Green, M. (1988). Towards rational drug scheduling. In J. Blackwell & P. Erickson (Eds.), *Illicit drugs in Canada* (pp. 186–208). Toronto: Nelson.

Greider, K. (1995). Quieting the crack-kid alarm. *The Drug Policy Letter, 27*, 16–17, 20–21.

Griffiths, C., & Verdun-Jones, S. (1989). *Canadian criminal justice*. Vancouver: Butterworths.

Gupta, T. (1995). Families of Native peoples, immigrants, and people of colour. In N. Mandell & A. Duffy (Eds.), *Canadian families* (pp. 141–174). Toronto: Harcourt Brace.

Gusfield, J. (1963). *Symbolic crusade: Status politics and the American temperance movement*. Urbana, IL: University of Illinois Press.

Hadaway, P., & Beyerstein, B. (1987). Then they came for the smokers but I didn't speak up because I wasn't a smoker: Legislation and tobacco use. *Canadian Psychology, 28*(3), 259–265.

Hadaway, P., Beyerstein, B., & Youdale, J. (1991). Canadian drug policies: Irrational, futile and unjust. *Journal of Drug Issues, 21*(1), 183–197.

Hagedorn, J. (1994). Homeboys, dope fiends, legits, and new jacks. *Criminology, 32*(2), 197–219.

Handwerker, L. (1994). Medical risk: Implicating poor pregnant women. *Social Science Medicine, 38*(5), 665–675.

Hanson, B., Beschner, G., Walters, J., & Bovelle, E. (Eds.). (1985). *Life with heroin: Voices from the inner city*. Toronto: Lexington Books.

Hansson, D. (1995). Agenda-ing gender: Feminism and the engendering of academic criminology in South Africa. In N. Rafter & F. Heidensohn (Eds.), *International feminist perspectives in criminology: Engendering a discipline* (pp. 39–60). Buckingham: Open University Press.

Harvey, L. (1990). *Critical social research*. London: Unwin Hyman.

Haskett, M., Miller, J., Whitworth, J., & Huffman, J. (1992). Intervention with cocaine-abusing mothers. *Families in Society: The Journal of Contemporary Human Services, 73*(25), 451–462.

Hawley, T., & Disney, E. (1992). Crack's children: The consequences of maternal cocaine abuse. *Social Policy Report, 11*(4), 1–23.

Health and Welfare Canada. (1991). *1990 narcotic, controlled and restricted drug statistics-analysis report*. Ottawa: Ministry of Supply and Services.

Henderson, S. (1993a). Luvdup and de-elited: Responses to drug use in the second decade. In P. Aggleton, P. Davies, & G. Hart (Eds.), *Aids: Facing the second decade* (pp. 119–130). London: Falmer.

Henderson, S. (1993b). Time for a make-over. *Druglink, 8*(5), 14–16.

Hepburn, M. (1990). Social problems. *Baillière's Clinical Obstetrics and Gynaecology, 4*(1), 149–168.

Hepburn, M. (1993a). Drug misuse in pregnancy. *Current Obstetrics & Gynaecology, 3*, 54–58.

Hepburn, M. (1993b). Drug use in pregnancy. *British Journal of Hospital Medicine, 49*(1), 51–55.

Higgins, A., Moxley, J., Pencharz, P., Mikolainis, D., & Dubois, S. (1989). Impact of the Higgins Nutrition Intervention Program on birth weight: A within-mother analysis. *Journal of the American Dietetic Association, 89*(8), 1097–1103.

hooks, b. (1989). *Talking back*. Boston: South End.

hooks, b. (1992). *Black looks: Race and representation*. Boston: South End.

Howard, J., Beckwith, L., Rodning, C., & Kropenske, V. (1989). The development of young children of substance-abusing parents: Insights from seven years of intervention and research. *Zero to Three, 9*(5), 8–12.

Humphries, D. (1993). Crack mothers, drug wars, and the politics of resentment. In K. Tunnell (Ed.), *Political crime in contemporary America* (pp. 31–48). New York: Garland.

Humphries, D., Dawson, J., Cronin, V., Keating, P., Wisniewski, C., & Eichfield, J. (1992). Mothers and children, drugs and crack: Reactions to maternal drug dependency. In C. Feinman (Ed.), *The criminalization of a woman's body* (pp. 203–221). New York: Haworth.

Hunt, D. (1974). Parental permissiveness as perceived by the offspring and the degree of marijuana usage among offspring. *Human Relations, 27*(3), 267–285.

Inciardi, J., Lockwood, D., & Pottieger, A. (1993). *Women and crack-cocaine*. Toronto: Maxwell Macmillan.

Institute for the Study of Drug Dependence (ISDD). (1992). *Drugs, pregnancy & childcare*. London: Author.

Irwin, K. (1995). Ideology, pregnancy and drugs: Differences between crack-cocaine, heroin and methamphetamine users. *Contemporary Drug Problems, 22*, 613–638.

Jackson, B. (1987). Rapport. In *Fieldwork* (pp. 68–78). Urbana IL: University of Illinois Press.

Jackson, M., & Berry, G. (1994). Motherhood and drug-dependency: The attributes of full-time versus part-time responsibility for child care. *International Journal of the Addictions, 29*(12), 1519–1535.

Jaffe, J.H. (1985). Drug addiction and drug abuse. In A.G. Gilman, L. Goodman, & A. Gilman (Eds.), *Goodman and Gilman's the pharmacological basis of therapeutics* (7th ed., pp. 532–581). New York: Macmillan.

Jaudes, P., Ekwo, E., & Voorhis, J. (1995). Association of drug abuse and child abuse. *Child Abuse & Neglect, 19*(9), 1065–1075.

Jayaratne, T.E., & Stewart, A.J. (1991). Quantitative and qualitative methods in the social sciences: Current feminist issues and practical strategies. In M.M. Fonow & J.A. Cook (Eds.), *Beyond methodology: Feminist scholarship as lived research* (pp. 85–106). Bloomington: Indiana University Press.

Johns, J., Noonan, L., Zimmerman, L., & Pedersen, C. (1994). Effects of chronic and acute cocaine treatment on the onset of maternal behavior and aggression in Sprague-Dawley rats. *Behavioral Neuroscience, 108*(1), 107–112.

Johnson, H., & Rodgers, K. (1993). A statistical overview of women and crime in Canada. In E. Adelberg & C. Currie (Eds.), *In conflict with the law* (pp. 95–116). Vancouver: Press Gang.

Judson, H.F. (1973). *Heroin addiction in Britain.* New York: Harcourt Brace Jovanovich.

Julien, R. (1992). *A primer of drug action* (6th ed.). New York: W.H. Freeman.

Kaltenbach, K., & Finnegan, L. (1989). Prenatal narcotic exposure: Perinatal and developmental effects. *Neurotoxicology, 10*(3), 597–604.

Kantor, G. (1978). Addicted mother, addicted baby – a challenge to health care providers. *American Journal of Maternal Child Nursing, 3,* 281–289.

Kaplan, E. (1994). Look who's talking, indeed: Fetal images in recent North American visual culture. In E. Glenn, G. Chang, & L. Forcey (Eds.), *Mothering: Ideology, experience, and agency* (pp. 121–137). New York: Routledge.

Kasinsky, R. (1994). Child neglect and 'unfit' mothers: Child savers in the progressive era and today. *Women & Criminal Justice, 6*(1), 97–129.

Kasl, C. (1992). *Many roads, one journey.* New York: Harper Perennial.

Kaye, K., Elkind, L., Goldberg, D., & Tytun, A. (1989). Birth outcomes for infants of drug-abusing mothers. *New York State Journal of Medicine, 89*(5), 256–261.

Kearney, M., Murphy, S., & Rosenbaum, M. (1994). Mothering on crack cocaine: A grounded theory analysis. *Social Science and Medicine, 38*(2), 351–361.

King, P. (1989). Should Mom be constrained in the best interests of the fetus? *Nova Law Review, 13,* 393–402.

Kirby, S., & McKenna, K. (1989). *Experience, research, social change: Methods from the margins.* Toronto: Garamond.

Kitzinger, S. (1992). *Ourselves as mothers.* Toronto: Bantam.

Klee, H., & Lewis, S. (1994, March). *Illicit drug use, pregnancy and childbirth.* Paper presented at the 5th International Conference on the Reduction of Drug-Related Harm, Toronto, Canada.

Knight, K., Rosenbaum, M., Kelley, M., Irwin, J., Washburn, A., & Wenger, L. (1996). Defunding the poor: The impact of lost access to subsidized methadone maintenance treatment on women injection drug users. *Journal of Drug Issues, 26*(4), 923–942.

Kolder, V., Gallagher, J., & Parsons, M. (1987). Court-ordered obstetrical interventions. *The New England Journal of Medicine, 316*(19), 1192–1196.

Koren, G. (1997). *The children of Neverland: The silent human disaster.* Toronto: The Kid In Us.

Koren, G., Graham, K., Shear, H., & Einarson, T. (1989). Bias against the null hypothesis: The reproductive hazards of cocaine. *The Lancet, 2*(8677), pp. 1440–1442.

LaPrairie, C. (1987). Native women and crime in Canada: A theoretical model. In E. Adelberg & C. Currie (Eds.), *Too few to count: Canadian women in conflict with the law* (pp. 103–112). Vancouver, BC: Press Gang.

Latchem, S. (1994). Antenatal care for drug users. *Midirs Midwifery Digest, 4*(4), 486–488.

Lauridsen-Hoegh, P. (1991). Caring for chemically dependent babies. *Nursing B.C., March,* 12–16.

Law Reform Commission of Canada. (1989). *Crimes against the foetus.* Ottawa: Author.

Lazarus, E. (1988). Poor women, poor outcomes: social class and reproductive health. In K. Michaelson (Ed.), *Childbirth in America: Anthropological perspectives* (pp. 39–54). South Hadley, MA: Bergin & Harvey.

Leeders, F. (1992). Drug-addicted parents and their children. *International Journal of Drug Policy, 3*(4), 204–210.

Lexchin, J. (1984). *The real pushers: A critical analysis of the Canadian drug industry.* Vancouver: New Star.

Lief, N. (1976). Some measures of parenting behavior for addicted and non-addicted mothers. In *Symposium on comprehensive health care for addicted families and their children* (pp. 38–47). Rockville, MD: National Institute on Drug Abuse.

Lifshitz, M., Wilson, G.S., Smith, E., & Desmond, M. (1983). Fetal and postnatal growth of children born to narcotic-dependent women. *Journal of Pediatrics, 102,* 686–691.

Lifshitz, M., Wilson, G.S., Smith, E., & Desmond, M. (1985). Factors affecting head growth and intellectual function in children of drug addicts. *Journal of Pediatrics, 75,* 269–274.

Lindenberg, C., Alexander, E., Gendrop, S., Nencioli, M., & Williams, D. (1991). A review of the literature on cocaine abuse in pregnancy. *Nursing Research, 40*(2), 69–75.

Lindesmith, A. (1947). *Opiate addiction.* Evanston, IL: Principia.

Lindesmith, A. (1965). *The addict and the law.* Bloomington: Indiana University Press.

Lofland, J., & Lofland, L.H. (1984). *Analyzing social settings: A guide to qualitative observation and analysis* (2nd ed.). Belmont, CA: Wadsworth.

Logli, P. (1990). Drugs in the womb: The newest battlefield in the war on drugs. *Criminal Justice Ethics, 9*(1), 23–39.

Lowe, J., & Ehrhard-Wingard, D. (1994, June). *Help and healing during withdrawal.* Paper presented at Conference on Effects of Alcohol and Other Drugs in Pregnancy: Issues for Families and Communities, Vancouver, BC.

Lowman, J. (1991). Prostitution in Canada. In M. Jackson & C. Griffiths (Eds.), *Canadian criminology: Perspectives on crime and criminality* (pp. 113–134). Toronto: Harcourt Brace Jovanovich.

Lowman, J., & Fraser, L. (1995). *Violence against persons who prostitute: The experience in British Columbia.* Department of Justice Canada.

MacKinnon, C. (1987). *Feminism unmodified: Discourses on life and law.* Cambridge, MA: Harvard University Press.

MacKinnon, M. (Ed.). (1991). *Each small step.* Charlottetown, PEI: gynergy.

Maher, L. (1992). Punishment and welfare: Crack cocaine and the regulation of mothering. In C. Feinman (Ed.), *The criminalization of a women's body* (pp. 157–192). New York: Haworth.

Maher, L. (1995). *Dope girls: Gender, race and class in the drug economy.* Unpublished doctoral dissertation, Rutgers, The State University of New Jersey, Newark.

Maier, K. (1992). *Forced cesarean section as reproductive control and violence: A feminist social work perspective on the 'Baby R' Case.* Unpublished master's thesis, Simon Fraser University, Burnaby, BC.

Mandell, N. (1995). Family histories. In N. Mandell & A. Duffy (Eds.), *Canadian families* (pp. 17–43). Toronto: Harcourt Brace.

Mariner, W., Glantz, L., & Annas, G. (1990). Pregnancy, drugs, and the perils of prosecution. *Criminal Justice Ethics, 9*(1), 30–39.

Martel, A. (1994). Policing aboriginal communities: Progress and pitfalls. In D. Currie and B. MacLean (Eds.), *Social inequality, social justice* (pp. 43–55). Vancouver: Collective.

Martin, D. (1991). *Passing the buck: Prosecution of welfare fraud; preservation of stereotypes.* Unpublished manuscript, Osgoode Hall Law School, York University, North York, ON.

Martin, D. (1992). The midwife's tale: Old wisdom and a new challenge to the control of reproduction. *Columbia Journal of Gender and Law, 3*(1), 417–448.

Martin, E. (1987). *The woman in the body: A cultural analysis of reproduction.* Boston: Beacon.

Martin, S., & Coleman, M. (1995). Judicial intervention in pregnancy. *McGill Law Review, 40,* 947–991.

Masson, K.M. (1992). *Familial ideology in the courts: The sentencing of women.* Unpublished master's thesis, Simon Fraser University, Burnaby, BC.

Mastrogiannis, D., Decavalas, G., Verma, U., & Tejani, N. (1990). Perinatal outcome after recent cocaine usage. *Obstetrics & Gynecology, 76*(1), 8–11.

Matthews, L. (1993). Outreach on the front line. *Druglink, 8*(2), 14–15.

Matthews, L.C.B., Dawes, G., Nadeau, B., Wong, L., & Alexander, B. (1995). *The British Columbia Key Informant Study.* Unpublished manuscript, Simon Fraser University, Burnaby, BC.

Mayes, L., Granger, R., Bornstein, M., & Zuckerman, B. (1992). The problem of prenatal cocaine exposure. *Journal of the American Medical Association, 267*(3), 406–408.

McDermott, P., & McBride, W. (1993). Crew 2000: Peer coalition in action. *Druglink, 8*(6), 13–15

McDonnell, K. (1986). Finding a common ground. In K. McDonnell (Ed.), *Adverse effects: Women and the pharmaceutical industry* (pp. 1–8). Toronto: Women's Educational Press.

McKenzie, D., Williams, B., & Single, E. (1997). *Canadian profile: Alcohol, tobacco & other drugs.* Toronto: Canadian Centre on Substance Abuse & The Addiction Research Foundation of Ontario.

McLaren, A. (1978). Birth control and abortion in Canada, 1870–1920. In A. Prentice & S. Trofimenkoff (Eds.), *The neglected majority: Essays in Canadian women's history* (Vol. 2, pp. 84–101). Toronto: McClelland & Stewart.

McLaren, A. (1990). *Our own master race.* Toronto: McClelland & Stewart.

Medrano, M. (1996). Does a discrete fetal solvent syndrome exist? *Alcoholism Treatment Quarterly, 14*(3), 59–76.

Merlo, A. (1993). Pregnant substance abusers: The new female offender. In R. Muraskin & T. Alleman (Eds.), *It's a crime: Women and justice* (pp. 146–158). Englewood Cliffs, NJ: Regents/Prentice-Hall.

Ministry for Children and Families. (1997). *Protocol for cooperation between staff ministry for children and families and physicians.* Victoria, BC: Author.

Ministry of Social Services. (1992/3). *Ministry of Social Services annual report* (pp. 20–23). Victoria, BC: Author.

Ministry of Social Services. (January, 1996). *Child, family and community service policy manual.* Victoria, BC: Author.

Mitchell, C. (1991). Introduction: A Canadian perspective on drug issues. *Journal of Drug Issues, 21*(1), 9–17.

Mitchell, T. (1996). Pre-natal protection? *Law Now, 21*(2), 7.

Mitchinson, W. (1988). The medical treatment of women. In S. Burt, L. Code, & L. Dorney (Eds.), *Changing patterns: Women in Canada* (pp. 237–263). Toronto: McClelland & Stewart.

Mitchinson, W. (1991). *The nature of their bodies.* Toronto: University of Toronto Press.

Mondanaro, J. (1989). *Chemically dependent women: assessment and treatment.* Lexington, MA: Lexington Books.

Monture, P. (1989). A vicious circle: Child welfare and the First Nations. *Canadian Journal of Women and the Law, 3*, 1–17.

Monture-Okanee, P., Thornhill, E., & Williams, T. (1993). After words. *Canadian Journal of Women and the Law, 6*(1), 224–233.

Morgan, J., & Zimmer, L. (1997). The social pharmacology of smokeable cocaine: Not all it's cracked up to be. In C. Reinarman & H. Levine (Eds.), *Crack in America: Demon drugs and social justice* (pp. 131–170). Berkeley: University of California Press.

Morgan, P. (1978). The legislation of drug law: Economic crisis and social control. *Journal of Drug Issues, 8*(1), 53–62.

Morgan, P. (1983). The political economy of drugs and alcohol: An introduction. *Journal of Drug Issues, 13*(1), 1–7.

Morgan, P., & Joe, K. (1997). Uncharted terrain: Contexts of experience among women in the illicit drug economy. *Women & Criminal Justice, 8*(3), 85–109.

Morgentaler, Smoling and Scott v. The Queen, 37 Canadian Criminal Cases (3d) 449–565.

Morris, R. (1985). Not the cause, nor the cure: Self image and control among inner-city black male heroin users. In B. Hanson et al. (Eds.), *Life with heroin: Voices from the inner city* (pp. 135–153). Toronto: Lexington Books.

Morrison, D., & Siney, C. (1996). A survey of the management of neonatal opiate withdrawal in England and Wales. *European Journal of Pediatrics, 155*(4), 323–326.

Murphy, J., Jellinek, M., Quinn, D., Smith, G., Poitrast, F., & Goshko, M. (1991). Substance abuse and serious child mistreatment: Prevalence, risk, and outcome in a court sample. *Child Abuse & Neglect, 15*, 197–211.

Musto, D.F. (1987). *The American disease: Origins of narcotic control* (Expanded ed.). New Haven, CT: Yale University Press.

Myers, B., Olson, H., & Kaltenbach, K. (1992). Cocaine-exposed infants: Myths and misunderstandings. *Zero to Three, 13*(1), 1–5.

Naeye, R.L., Branc, W., Leblanc, W., & Khatamee, M.A. (1973). Fetal complications of maternal heroin addiction: Abnormal growth, infections and episodes of stress. *Journal of Pediatrics, 83*, 1065–1061.

Noble, A. (1997). Is prenatal drug use child abuse? Reporting practices and coerced treatment in California. In P. Erickson, D. Riley, Y. Cheung, & P. O'Hare (Eds.), *Harm reduction: A new direction for drug policies and programs* (pp. 174–191). Toronto: University of Toronto Press.

Nsiah-Jefferson, L. (1989). Reproductive law, women of color, and low-income women. In S. Cohen & N. Taub (Eds.), *Reproductive laws for the 1990's* (pp. 23–67). Clifton, NJ: Human Press.

Nugent, J. (1994). Cross-cultural studies of child development: Implications for clinicians. *Zero to Three, 15*(2), 1–8.

Nulman, I., Rovet, J., Altmann, D., Bradley, C., Einarson, T., & Koren, G. (1994). Neurodevelopment of adopted children exposed in utero to cocaine. *Canadian Medical Association Journal, 151*(11), 1591–1597.

Oakley, A. (1984). *The captured womb.* Oxford: Blackwell.

Oakley, A. (1986). Feminism, motherhood and medicine – who cares? In J. Mitchell & A. Oakley (Eds.), *What is feminism?* (pp. 127–150). Oxford: Blackwell.

Oakley, A. (1992). *Social support and motherhood.* Oxford: Blackwell.

O'Hare, P. (1992). A note on the concept of harm reduction. In P. O'Hare, R. Newcombe, A. Matthews, E.C. Buning, & E. Drucker (Eds.), *The reduction of drug-related harm* (pp. xiii–xvii). New York: Routledge.

O'Hare, P. (1994). 'Starring harm reduction.' *International Journal of Drug Policy, 5*(3), 199–200.

Orme, T., & Rimmer, J. (1981). Alcoholism and child abuse: A review. *Journal of Studies on Alcohol, 42*(3), 273–287.

Paltrow, L. (1992). *Criminal prosecutions against pregnant women.* Reproductive Freedom Project. New York: American Civil Liberties Union Foundation.

Pawl, J. (1992). Interventions to strengthen relationships between infants and drug-abusing or recovering parents. *Zero to Three, 13*(1), 6–10.

Peak, K., & Papa, F. (1993). Criminal justice enters the womb: Enforcing the 'right to be born drug-free.' *Journal of Criminal Justice, 21*, 245–263.

Pearce, D. (1990). Welfare is not for women: Why the war on poverty cannot conquer the feminization of poverty. In L. Gordon (Ed.), *Women, the state, and welfare* (pp. 265–279). Madison: University of Wisconsin Press.

Peele, S. (1989). *Diseasing of America: Addiction treatment out of control.* Toronto: Lexington Books.

Peele, S., & Brodsky, A. (1991). *The truth about addiction and recovery.* New York: Simon & Schuster.

Penfold, P.S., & Walker, G.A. (1983). *Women and the psychiatric paradox.* Montreal: Eden Press.

Perry, L. (1979). *Women and drug use: An unfeminine dependency.* London: Institute for the Study of Drug Dependency.

Petchesky, R. (1990). *Abortion and woman's choice.* Boston: Northeastern University Press.

Peterson, L., Gable, S., & Saldana, L. (1996). Treatment of maternal addiction to prevent child abuse and neglect. *Addictive Behaviors, 21*(6), 789–801.

Preble, E., & Casey, J.J. (1969). Taking care of business. *International Journal of the Addictions, 4*, 2.

Pulkingham, J. (1994). Private troubles, private solutions: Poverty among divorced women and the politics of support enforcement and child custody determination. *Canadian Journal of Law and Society, 9*(2), 73–97.

Radford, L. (1987). Legalising woman abuse. In J. Hanmer & M. Maynard (Eds.), *Women, violence and social control* (pp. 135–151). London: Macmillan.

Re 'Baby R' (1988) 15 R.F.L. 225 (B.C.S.C.).

Re 'Children's Aid Society of City of Belleville, Hastings County and T et al' (1987) 59 O.R. (2d) 204 (Ont. Prov. Ct.).

Re 'Children's Aid Society for the District of Kenora and J.L.' (1981) 134 D.L.R. (3d) 249 (Ont. Prov. Ct. Fam. Div.).

Re *'Winnipeg Child and Family Services (Northwest Area) v. G.'* (1997).

Reed, B. (1987). Developing women-sensitive drug dependence treatment services: Why so difficult?. *Journal of Psychoactive Drugs, 19*(2), 151–164.

Reinarman, C. (1979). Moral entrepreneurs and political economy: Historical and ethnographic notes on the construction of the cocaine menace. *Contemporary Crises, 3,* 225–254.

Reinharz, S. (1992). *Feminist methods in social research.* New York: Oxford University Press.

Rementeria, J., & Nunag, N. (1973). Narcotic withdrawal in pregnancy: Stillbirth incidence with a case report. *American Journal of Obstetrics and Gynaecology, 116*(8), 1152–1156.

Rempel, J. (1989). Letters to the editors. *Zero to Three, 9*(5), 23–24.

Report of the Aboriginal Committee (1992). *Liberating our children, liberating our nations.* Victoria, BC: Ministry of Social Services.

Rich, A. (1986). *Of woman born* (10th ed.). New York: Norton.

Roberts, D. (1996, October 19). Solvent-abuse case to go to Supreme Court. *The Globe and Mail,* pp. A1, A2.

Robertson J. (1989). Reconciling offspring and maternal interests during pregnancy. In S. Cohen & N. Taub (Eds.), *Reproductive laws for the 1990s* (pp. 259–274). Clifton, NJ: Humana.

Robins, L. (1966). *Deviant children growing up.* Boston: Williams & Wilkins.

Robins, L., & Mills, J. (Eds.). (1993). Effects of in utero exposure to street drugs. *American Journal of Public Health, 83* (Suppl.), 1–32.

Robin-Vergeer, B. (1990). The problem of the drug-exposed newborn: A return to principled intervention. *Standard Law Review, 42*(3), 745–809.

Rodgers, R., & Mitchell, C. (1991). *Mental health experts and the criminal courts.* Scarborough, ON: Carswell.

Rogers, J., & Buffalo, M. (1974). Fighting back: Nine models of adaptation to a deviant label. *Social Problems, 22*(1), 101–118.

Rosenbaum, M. (1981). *Women on heroin.* New Brunswick, NJ: Rutgers University Press.

Rosenbaum, M., & Murphy, S. (1987). Not the picture of health: Women on methadone. *Journal of Psychoactive Drugs, 19*(2), 217–226.

Rosenbaum, M., Murphy, S., Irwin, J., & Watson, L. (1990). Women and crack: What's the real story? *The Drug Policy Letter, 11*(2), 2–6.

Rothman, B. (1989). Motherhood: Beyond patriarchy. *Nova Law Review, 13,* 481–484.

Royal Commission on New Reproductive Technologies. (1993). *Proceed with care: Final report of the Royal Commission on New Reproductive Technologies.* Ottawa: Minister of Government Services.

Rudd, A., & Taylor, D. (Eds.). (1992). *Voices of women living with AIDS.* Toronto: Second Story.

Russell, S.A., & Wilsnack, S. (1991). Adult survivors of child sexual abuse: Substance abuse and other consequences. In P. Roth (Ed.), *Alcohol and drugs are women's issues.* Vol. I: *A review of the issues* (pp. 61–70). Metuchen, NJ: Women's Action Alliance & The Scarecrow Press.

Sandmaier, M. (1980). *The invisible alcoholics.* New York: McGraw-Hill.

Saxell, L. (1994). *Perceptions of risk: Women's and midwives' experience of nulliparous pregnancy over 35.* Unpublished master's thesis, Thames Valley University, London, England.

Schur, E.M. (1962). *Narcotic addiction in Britain and America: The impact of public policy.* Bloomington: Indiana University Press.

Segura, D. (1994). Working at motherhood: Chicana and Mexican immigrant mothers and employment. In E. Glenn, G. Chang, & L. Forcey (Eds.), *Mothering: Ideology, experience, and agency* (pp. 211–233). New York: Routledge.

Seldin, N. (1972). The family of the addict: A review of the literature. *International Journal of the Addictions, 7*(1), 97–107.

Shaver, F. (1993). Prostitution: A female crime? In E. Adelberg & C. Currie (Eds.), *In conflict with the law* (pp. 153–173). Vancouver: Press Gang.

Shaw, M. (1985). Should child abuse laws be extended to include fetal abuse? In A. Milunsky & G. Annas (Eds.), *Genetics and the law III* (pp. 310–315). New York: Plenum.

Shaw, S. (1994). Mothering under slavery in the antebellum South. In E. Glenn, G. Chang, & L. Forcey (Eds.), *Mothering: Ideology, experience, and agency* (pp. 237–258). New York: Routledge.

Shoham, S., & Hoffman, J. (1991). *A primer in the sociology of crime.* New York: Harrow & Heston.

Simpson, S. (1989). Feminist theory, crime and justice. *Criminology, 27*(4), 605–631.

Siney, C. (1994). Team effort helps pregnant drug users. *Midirs Midwifery Digest, 4*(2), 229–231.

Siney, C. (Ed.). (1995). *The pregnant addict.* Cheshire, UK: Books for Midwives.

Siney, C., Kidd, M., Walkinshaw, S., Morrison, C., & Manasse, P. (1995). Opiate dependency in pregnancy. *British Journal of Midwifery, 3*(2), 69–73.

Small, S. (1978). Canadian narcotics legislation, 1908–1923: A conflict model interpretation. In W. Greenaway & S. Brickey (Eds.), *Law and social control in Canada* (pp. 28–42). Scarborough, ON: Prentice-Hall.

Smart, C. (1989). *Feminism and the power of law.* London: Routledge.

Smart, C., & Smart, B. (1978). Women and social control: An introduction. In C. Smart & B. Smart (Eds.), *Women, sexuality and social control* (pp. 1–7). London: Routledge & Kegan Paul.

Smith, D. (1986). Institutional ethnography: A feminist method. *Resources for Feminist Research, 15*(1), 6–13.

Solinger, R. (1994). Race and 'value': Black and white illegitimate babies, 1945–1965. In N. Glenn, G. Chang, & L. Forcey (Eds.), *Mothering: Ideology, experience, and agency* (pp. 287–310). New York: Routledge.

Solomon, R. (1988). Canada's federal drug legislation. In J. Blackwell & P. Erickson (Eds.), *Illicit drugs in Canada* (Pre-publication ed., pp. 117–129). Toronto: Methuen.

Solomon, R., & Green, M. (1988). The first century: The history of nonmedical opiate use and control policies in Canada, 1870–1970. In J. Blackwell & P. Erickson (Eds.), *Illicit drugs in Canada* (Pre-publication ed., pp. 88–116). Toronto: Methuen.

Sowder, B., & Burt, M. (1980). Children of addicts and nonaddicts: A comparative investigation in five urban sites. In *Heroin-addicted parents and their children: Two reports.* (National Institute on Drug Abuse Services Research Report, pp. 19–35). Washington, DC: U.S. Department of Health and Human Services; Public Health Service; Alcohol, Drug Abuse, and Mental Health Administration.

Stanley, L., & Wise, S. (1979). Feminist research, feminist consciousness and experiences of sexism. *Women's Studies International Quarterly, 2*, 359–374.

Steinberg, D. (1994). Pregnancy, drugs and the law. *Contemporary ob/gyn, 3*(4), 10–17.

Steele, B. (1987). Psychodynamic factors in child abuse. In R. Helfer & R. Kempe (Eds.). *The battered child* (4th edition, pp. 81–114), Chicago: University of Chicago Press.

Stephenson, P., & Wagner, M. (1993). Reproductive rights and the medical care system: A plea for rational health policy. *Journal of Public Health Policy, 14*(2), 174–181.

Sterk-Elifson, C. (1996). Just for fun? Cocaine use among middle-class women. *Journal of Drug Issues, 26*(1), 63–76.

Stern, R. (1966). The pregnant addict. *American Journal of Obstetrics and Gynaecology, 94*(2), 253–257.

Stevenson, G., Lingley, L., Trasov, G., & Stansfield, H. (1956). *Drug addiction in British Columbia: A research survey.* Unpublished manuscript, University of British Columbia, Vancouver, BC.

Stoddart, K. (1982). The enforcement of narcotics violations in a Canadian city: Heroin users' perspectives on the production of official statistics. *Canadian Journal of Criminology, 24*, 425–438.

Stone, M., Salerno, L., Green, M., & Zelson, C. (1971). Narcotic addiction in pregnancy. *American Journal of Obstetrics and Gynaecology, 109*(5), 716–723.

Strauss, A.L., & Corbin, J. (1990). *Basics of qualitative research: Grounded theory procedures and techniques*. Newbury Park, CA: Sage.

Streissguth, A., Grant, T., Ernst, C., & Phipps, P. (1994, June). *Reaching out to the highest risk mothers: The birth to 3 project* (Tech. Rep. no. 94-12). Seattle: University of Washington, Fetal Alcohol & Drug Unit.

Sunny Hill Hospital for Children. (1992a). *NAS Program clinical manifestations of withdrawal*. Vancouver, BC: Author.

Sunny Hill Hospital for Children. (1992b). *NAS Program follow-up instruction*. Vancouver, BC: Author.

Sunny Hill Hospital for Children. (1992c). *Potential long-term NAS problems*. Vancouver, BC: Author.

Sunny Hill Hospital Tertiary Task Force. (1993). *NAS/FAS Task Force final report*. Vancouver, BC: Ministry of Health, Tertiary Task Force on NAS/FAS.

Szasz, T.S. (1974). *Ceremonial chemistry: The ritual persecution of drugs, addicts, and pushers*. New York: Anchor.

Tait, K. (1996, February 5). Addiction, parenting mutually exclusive. *The Province*, p. A14.

Taylor, A. (1993). *Women drug users*. Oxford: Clarendon Press.

Thane, P. (1978). Women and the Poor Law in Victorian and Edwardian England. *History Workshop: A Journal of Socialist Historians, 6*(2), 227–232.

Theidon, K. (1995). Taking a hit: Pregnant drug users and violence. *Contemporary Drug Problems, 22*, 663–686.

The People's Law School. (1993). *Welfare appeals*. Vancouver, BC: Author.

Thurer, S. (1994). *The myths of motherhood*. New York: Houghton Mifflin.

Tittle, B., & St. Claire, N. (1989). Promoting the health and development of drug-exposed infants through a comprehensive clinic model. *Zero to Three, 9*(5), 18–20.

Trebach, A.S. (1982). *The heroin solution*. New Haven, CT: Yale University Press.

Trebach, A.S. (1987). *The great drug war*. New York: Macmillan.

Tunnell, K. (Ed.). (1993). *Political crime in contemporary America*. New York: Garland.

Turpel, M.E. (1993). Patriarchy and paternalism: The legacy of the Canadian state for First Nations women. *Canadian Journal of Women and the Law, 6*(1), 174–192.

Vernotica, E., Lisciotto, C., Rosenblatt, J., & Morrell, J. (1996). Cocaine transiently impairs maternal behavior in the rat. *Behavioral Neuroscience, 110*(2), 315–323.

Wagner, M. (1994). *Pursuing the birth machine*. Camperdown, Australia: ACE Graphics.

Waldorf, D. (1973). *Careers in dope*. Englewood Cliffs, NJ: Prentice-Hall.

Waldorf, D., & Biernacki, P. (1979). Natural recovery from heroin addiction. *Journal of Drug Issues, 9*(2), 281–289.

Waldorf, D., Murphy, S., Reinarman, C., & Joyce, B. (1977). *Doing coke: An ethnography of cocaine users and sellers*. Washington, DC: Drug Abuse Council.

Waldorf, D., & Reinarman, C. (1975). Addicts – everything but human beings. *Urban Life, 4*(1), 30–53.

Waldorf, D., Reinarman, C., & Murphy, S. (1991). *Cocaine changes*. Philadelphia: Temple University Press.

Walters, J. (1985). 'Taking care of business' updated: A fresh look at the daily routine of the heroin user. In B. Hanson et al. (Eds.), *Life with heroin: Voices from the inner city* (pp. 31–48). Toronto: Lexington Books.

Weil, A. (1972) *The natural mind*. Boston: Houghton Mifflin.

Weil, A., & Rosen, W. (1993). *Chocolate to morphine: Understanding mind-active drugs*. Boston: Houghton Mifflin.

Wellisch, D., & Steinberg, M. (1980). Parenting attitudes of addict mothers. *The International Journal of the Addictions, 15*(6), 809–819.

Weston, D., Ivins, B., Zuckerman, B., Jones, C., & Lopez, R. (1989). Drug-exposed babies: Research and clinical issues. *Zero to Three, 9*(5), 1–7.

White, E. (1992). Foster parenting the drug-affected baby. *Zero to Three, 13*(1), 13–17.

Wijngaart, G. (1991). *Competing perspectives on drug use: The Dutch experience*. Amsterdam: Swets & Zeitlinger.

Williams, K., & Bruce, L. (1994). Drug abuse in pregnancy. *Journal of the Society of Obstetricians and Gynaecologists of Canada, 16*(3), 1469–1476.

Williams-Peterson, M., Myers, B., Degen, H., Knisely, J., Elswichk, R., & Schnoll, S. (1994). Drug-using and nonusing women: Potential for child abuse, child-rearing attitudes, social support, and affection for expected baby. *International Journal of the Addictions, 29*(12), 1631–1643.

Winick, C. (1962). Maturing out of narcotic addiction. *Bulletin on Narcotics, 14*(1), 1–7.

Winnicott, D. (1987). *Babies and their mothers*. New York: Addison-Wesley.

Wisotsky, S. (1986). *Breaking the impasse in the war on drugs*. New York: Greenwood.

Wong, S. (1994). Diverted mothering: Representations of caregivers of color in the age of 'multiculturalism.' In E. Glenn, G. Chang, & L. Forcey (Eds.), *Mothering: Ideology, experience, and agency* (pp. 67–91). New York: Routledge.

Zarin-Ackerman, J. (1976). Developmental assessment of all infants born to the family care program. In *Symposium on comprehensive health care for addicted families and their children* (pp. 99–106). Rockville, MD: National Institute on Drug Abuse.

Zinberg, N., & Harding, W. (1979). Control and intoxicant use: A theoretical and practical overview. *Journal of Drug Issues, 9*(2), 121–143.

Zinberg, N., Harding, W., & Apsler, R. (1978). What is drug abuse? *Journal of Drug Issues, 8*(1), 9–35.

Index

Da'